Physician Alignment and Compensation Models: The Second Generation

Max Reiboldt, CPA
Justin Chamblee, MAcc, CPA
Ellis M. "Mac" Knight, MD, MBA
COKER GROUP

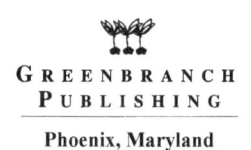

GREENBRANCH
PUBLISHING

Phoenix, Maryland

Copyright © 2017 by Greenbranch Publishing, LLC
ISBN: 978-0-9984985-4-6
eISBN: 978-0-9984985-5-3

PO Box 208
Phoenix, MD 21131
Phone: (800) 933-3711
Fax: (410) 329-1510
Email: info@greenbranch.com
Websites: www.greenbranch.com, www.mpmnetwork.com, www.soundpractice.net

All rights reserved. No part of this book shall be reproduced, stored in a retrieval system, or transmitted by any means, i.e., electronic, mechanical, photocopying, recording, or otherwise, without written permission of the publisher. Please do not participate in or encourage piracy of copyrighted materials in violation of the authors' rights. Purchase only authorized editions. Routine photocopying or electronic distribution to others is a copyright violation. Please notify us immediately at (800) 933-3711 if you have received any unauthorized editorial from this book.

No patent liability is assumed with respect to the use of the information contained herein. Although every precaution has been taken in the preparation of this book, the publisher and the authors assume no responsibility for errors or omissions. Nor is any liability assumed from damages resulting from the use of the information contained herein. For information, contact Greenbranch Publishing, PO Box 208, Phoenix, MD 21131.

This book includes representations of the author's personal experiences and do not reflect actual patients or medical situations.

This book is not intended as a substitute for the medical advice of physicians. The reader should regularly consult a physician in matters relating to his/her health and particularly with respect to any symptoms that may require diagnosis or medical attention.

The strategies contained herein may not be suitable for every situation. This publication is designed to provide general medical practice management information and is sold with the understanding that neither the author nor the publisher is engaged in rendering legal, accounting, ethical, or clinical advice. If legal or other expert advice is required, the services of a competent professional person should be sought.

Greenbranch Publishing books are available at special quantity discounts for bulk purchases as premiums, fund-raising, or educational use. Contact info@greenbranch.com or (800) 933-3711.

13   8 7 6 5 4 3 2 1

Copyedited, typeset, indexed, and printed in the United States of America

PUBLISHER
Nancy Collins

EDITORIAL ASSISTANT
Jennifer Weiss

BOOK DESIGNER
Laura Carter
Carter Publishing Studio

COPYEDITOR
Pat George

Table of Contents

About the Authors iv
Contributors vii
Acknowledgements x
Dedication xi
Introduction xiii

SECTION 1 1

CHAPTER 1: Overview of Compensation Plans 1

CHAPTER 2: Current First Generation Plans 11

CHAPTER 3: Market and Industry Dynamics Promoting New
Compensation Paradigms 23

CHAPTER 4: "Second" Generation Compensation Models 39

CHAPTER 5: Negotiating Second Generation Contracts 55

Appendix A 63

Appendix B 71

Appendix C 76

Appendix D 101

SECTION 2 117

CHAPTER 1: Overview of Stage I Alignment 117

CHAPTER 2: Market/Industry Dynamics Promoting Stage II
Alignment 133

CHAPTER 3: Stage II Alignment Models and Entities 145

CHAPTER 4: Structuring Stage II Alignment Models 157

CHAPTER 5: Implementation of Stage II Alignment Models 177

CHAPTER 6: Where Do We Go from Here with Value-Based
Structures and Strategies: Will There be a Stage III? 191

About the Authors

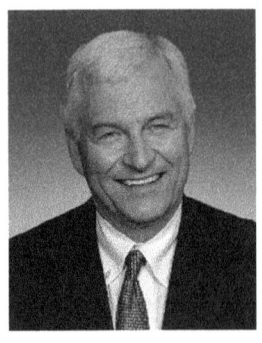

Max Reiboldt, CPA, is president/CEO of Coker Group with 44 years of total experience; the last 25 years specifically focused on healthcare. He has experienced first-hand the incredible changes of healthcare providers, which uniquely equips him to handle strategic, tactical, financial, and management issues that health systems and physicians face in today's evolving marketplace.

From his extensive work with health systems/hospitals, medical practices, and related healthcare entities, Mr. Reiboldt understands the nuances of the healthcare industry, especially in such a dynamic age. He understands healthcare organizations' needs to maintain viability in a highly-competitive market. His experience of having "experienced everything" in the healthcare industry equips him to provide pertinent counsel to clients. Whether a transitional provider or a more cutting-edge healthcare entity, Mr. Reiboldt is uniquely qualified to work with these organizations to provide sound solutions to every day and long-range challenges.

As president/CEO, Mr. Reiboldt oversees Coker Group's services and the general operations of the firm. His "first love" is working with clients, providing sound financial, strategic, and tactical solutions to hospitals and health systems, medical practices, and other healthcare entities through keen analysis and problem-solving. Working with organizations of all sizes, Reiboldt engages in consulting projects nationwide.

An avid writer and speaker, Reiboldt enjoys educating healthcare leaders through books, white papers, articles, and speaking at national symposiums. His expertise encompasses physician/hospital alignment initiatives, hospital service line development, clinical integration initiatives, financial analyses (including physician compensation plans), mergers and acquisitions, hospital and practice strategic planning, ancillary services development, PHO/IPA/MSO/CIN development, appraisals, and "accountable care era" consultation. As the industry moves to adapting to the many changes in response to healthcare reform, including the entire "volume-to-value" paradigm, he leads Coker Group's efforts in this arena.

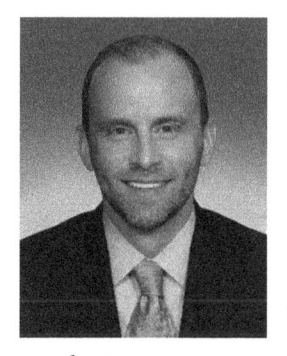

Justin Chamblee, MAcc, CPA, is a senior vice president and director of operations at Coker Group. As an executive healthcare consultant and certified public accountant, he provides strategic and financial counsel to healthcare organizations, physician practices, and healthcare attorneys throughout the country, dealing primarily with physician compensation and hospital-physician transactions. His work in physician compensation involves strategy, by assisting healthcare organizations to restructure their compensation arrangements to ensure they are consistent with the market on a macro and micro basis. Chamblee's work also involves compensation valuation, by helping healthcare organizations ensure that their financial arrangements comply with the requirements of fair market value and commercial reasonableness. Other areas of expertise include contract negotiations, sale/acquisition negotiations, strategic planning and business plan development, and other areas of finance.

As a recognized thought leader, Chamblee frequently presents at national conferences where physician leaders, healthcare legal counsel, and health system administrators gather to gain knowledge in the areas of physician compensation and hospital-physician integration. He has also authored several books and professional publications in collaboration with Greenbranch Publishing, Healthcare Financial Management Association, the American Medical Association, and HealthLeaders Media.

In addition to his consulting role, Mr. Chamblee is Coker's director of operations, directing the day-to-day functioning of the company.

He has a BBA in Accounting and a Master's in Accounting from Abilene Christian University, licensed as a Certified Public Accountant in the State of Texas, and a member of the American Institute of Certified Public Accountants. Additionally, he has completed extensive training through the Harvard Business School Leadership program.

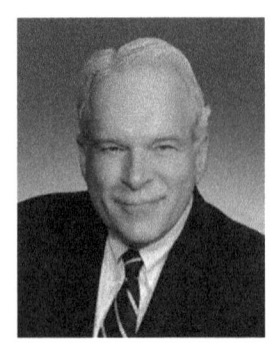

Ellis M. ("Mac") Knight, MD, MBA, FACP, FACHE, FHM, is senior vice president and chief medical officer of Coker Group. With over 30 years in the healthcare arena, he has developed significant experience and knowledge in this industry.

Before joining Coker, Dr. Knight served as the chief physician and clinical integration officer for Palmetto Health in Columbia, South Carolina. There, he oversaw Palmetto Health's employed physician network and helped to develop and manage their clinical integration program, The Palmetto Health Quality Collaborative. Earlier, he was Palmetto Health Richland's vice president for medical affairs.

Dr. Knight graduated from Stanford University with a Bachelor of Arts degree in Human Biology and received his doctor of medicine degree, cum laude, from the University of Oregon Health Science Center's School of Medicine. He earned a Master of Business Administration from the University of Massachusetts at Amherst. Mac holds fellowships in the American College of Physicians, the Society of Hospital Medicine, and the American College of Healthcare Executives.

Dr. Knight oversees Coker Group's hospital strategy and operations services and is Coker Group's chief medical officer. He has a particular interest and expertise in population health management, clinical care process design, cost accounting and hospital-physician integration.

Contributors

As a senior associate in Coker Group's Finance, Operations, and Strategy division, **Jessica Combs** engages in consulting projects with physicians and health systems nationwide. Jessica's career in healthcare consulting began in 2008 when she was hired by Coker to assist in the Community Needs Assessment (CNA) research and development process. She ensured accurate and realistic reporting and was responsible for the initial development of the CNA report and recommendations based on the statistical data available. After several years in this capacity, Jessica transitioned to the Finance, Operations, and Strategy division to participate in various fair market value reviews, compensation model development projects, physician-hospital alignment transactions, and financial analyses. Her work encompasses market research for tangible asset valuations, as well. Since 2014, Jessica also assists in the Practice Management Division. Recently, she engaged in a system-wide patient access optimization project for outpatient clinics affiliated with a prominent academic medical center. With a Bachelor of Science degree from Embry-Riddle Aeronautical University, her scientific background allows Jessica to think critically and strategically while assisting in the variety of assignments Coker entrusts to her.

Taylor Harrison, MBA, is an Associate Consultant with Coker's Financial and Hospital Operations services division. She works predominantly in the Financial and Alignment Services section, providing clients with consultative assistance for alignment and integration, financial analyses, accountable care responsiveness, and service line development. Taylor also assists in Coker's ValuePath service line, helping clients respond to value-based reimbursement changes and developing population health management strategies. Taylor recently worked on an acquisition for a large health system in the Southeast, coordinating a confirmatory diligence review.

Ms. Harrison comes with extensive experience in healthcare consulting, particularly in the hospital administration arena, such as credentialing and privileging management. She is a recent graduate of Terry College of Business at the University of Georgia with a degree in Business Management and is currently pursuing a Master's in Business Administration.

Jon Morris, J.D., MBA, is a manager with Coker Group. He works with clients on physician compensation compliance and strategy. The majority of his practice involves reviewing physician compensation arrangements, providing fair market value (FMV) and commercial reasonableness (CR) opinions, implementing best practices for physician compensation governance, and designing physician compensation plans that meet the client's strategic and financial goals.

Mr. Morris graduated from Alma College with a Bachelor of Business Administration degree followed by a Master's in Business Administration from Valparaiso University. Also at Valparaiso, he attained a Juris Doctorate.

Daniel W. Kiehl, J.D., Ll.M., is an associate consultant with Coker's finance operations strategy team. Daniel works on a myriad of assignments and Coker service lines. He also provides compliance consulting for both the Practice Management and the Financial/Operations/Strategy divisions. Daniel interfaces with current and prospective clients and internal team members on legal or regulatory compliance issues that are relevant to particular projects. Daniel performs a variety of services to include contract and regulation reviews and analysis and problem-solving. Daniel is an expert in matters relating to various legal, regulatory, political, ethical, and economic aspects of healthcare delivery.

Daniel comes to Coker Group with four years of experience as a litigation attorney. After graduating from Indiana State University, receiving a Bachelor of Science degree, Daniel went on to Valparaiso University School of Law in Valparaiso, Indiana, where he received his Juris Doctor. Daniel was awarded his Ll.M. degree in Health Law from Loyola University School of Law in August 2016.

Daniel is a member of the American Health Lawyers Association, the Health Care Compliance Association, and the Medical Group Management Association. He also served as a Non-Commissioned Officer in the United States Army Reserve and as an Intern for Congressman Brad Ellsworth in Washington, D.C.

Laura Ropski, MBA, MPH, is an Associate Consultant for Coker's Financial and Hospital Operations division. Laura performs a variety of services to include Financial Alignment, Hospital Operations, and

Strategic Services projects. She has a breadth of experience and exposure in various areas of healthcare consulting, including private practice and hospital systems in both financial advisory and operations/strategic services.

Laura graduated from Georgia College & State University with a Bachelor of Business Administration degree in Economics and Marketing. She also earned an MBA from the University of Georgia. Further, she holds a Master's of Public Health in Health Policy & Management from Emory University.

Acknowledgements

The combined knowledge and experience of a team with a common mission promises to yield a positive result when the assignment is worthy. In healthcare, the axiom could not be truer.

As consultant advisors, we appreciate the opportunity to share knowledge and experience through the capable staff at Greenbranch Publishing. Nancy Collins and her team are conduits of education and information to apprise healthcare leaders—physicians, health system executives, and administrators—of best business practices and sound financial management principles in the delivery of healthcare.

It is a privilege for Coker to team up with Greenbranch to share knowledge and experience.

Dedication

The authors and contributors dedicate this book to healthcare executives, administrators, and workers at every level in the healthcare spectrum. We recognize your frustration in the midst of continual change. It may seem that about the time you've nailed down a solution to a problem, as in the first generation compensation plans and integration models, the cosmos evolves to another galaxy. The confusion continues.

Nevertheless, you never give up. You forge ahead into the uncharted pathways in an unceasing effort to deliver the best healthcare you can provide. You race for quality, cost containment, and population health management in a fiercely competitive field.

We offer this book to help you journey through the current and forthcoming quandaries and challenges you will address. Our hope is that the information in these chapters will be helpful as you negotiate the nuances of the second generation of physician-hospital alignment and compensation models. Our goal is to guide your paths and give you confidence as you stay on track.

Introduction

The current era of healthcare affiliation among physicians, hospitals, other healthcare providers, and outside independent investors has been underway for 10 to 15 years. The latest "wave" of transactional relationships started around the turn of this century, and the result is that much has occurred and thousands of transactions have transpired.

Some people target March 2010 as the critical point that the new era began. That marked the date that President Obama signed the Affordable Care Act (ACA) legislation into law. While not a great deal happened immediately, a lot has occurred in the last two to three years, and conceivably, there is much more action to come. Even before the signing of the ACA into law, many events in the healthcare industry in the United States pulled hospitals and physicians and other healthcare providers together. Those relationships continue to develop but with additional elements such as the Medicare Access and CHIP Reauthorization Act of 2015 (MACRA) and the related Merit-Based Payment Incentive System (MIPS) and terms such as Alternative Payment Methodologies (APMs), clinically integrated networks (CINs), and other consortiums.

Given the length of time that these types of relations or affiliations have been in effect, many original contracts that formed the basis of these arrangements have or will soon expire. Thus, the appropriate term for the new deals is "second generation" transactions. One of the first questions our clients often ask as we provide advisory services to our broad base of healthcare providers, i.e., hospitals, physician groups, and others, is what happens with the renewal agreement (vis-à-vis second generation contract) when this one expires? The answers are myriad and warrant considerable discussion, review, and analysis. In the first section of this book, we discuss physician compensation models in both the first and now the second generation affiliations. We consider the compensation incentive plans that were implemented and worked reasonably well in those first generation affiliations. Now, however, as the contracts are coming up for renewal (e.g., second generation), we are finding significant variations in the need for all involved parties to respond to the changing reimbursement paradigm, often referenced as moving from "volume-to-value" reimbursement.

Another dynamic at play in this second generation model (as we discuss in this book) is whether the particular relationship has moved sufficiently away from fee-for-volume reimbursement to warrant significant changes in the compensation incentive structure. Usually, a hybrid model is developed that maintains a significant emphasis on volume-based reimbursement and incentives, but it also includes some considerations for quality, cost savings, and additional "value" based reimbursement incentives. Many of these models make allowances for the uncertainty of the future, meaning that if, in fact, the reimbursement paradigm changes substantially during the course of the next contract (second generation agreement), the compensation incentive structure will correspond accordingly.

Thus, the first section of this book drills down in some detail on both the first and now second generation compensation models.

Alignment initiatives have also experienced significant changes, and as they move to second generation agreements, we must consider the corresponding alternatives. By this we mean that the first generation alignment models could have been tied more so to limited or even moderate forms of affiliation, stopping short of "full" alignment. And many of those that did embark upon and complete full alignment initiatives are now looking beyond as they consider the Stage II options.

Primarily, the Stage II options are not just employment or professional services agreements (PSAs) or even clinical co-management (CCMA) models. They are now under consideration within the context of CINs and fully operative accountable care organizations (ACOs). We explore these "end-game" models in some detail in the second section of this book, drawing conclusions and offering recommendations for developing strategic and tactical options. In these discussions, we explore the usefulness and value, and peer into the proverbial crystal ball for the "look" of these Stage II clinically integrated models and potentially a Stage III vision.

This book considers a fair amount of history as we can learn from past occurrences, and we also explore, in some detail, the second generation compensation models and/or Stage II integration/alignment strategies and initiatives. We trust that the groundwork we lay will assist the readers of this book to develop their strategy for dealing with these critical issues, both now and in the future.

SECTION 1

CHAPTER 1

Overview of Compensation Plans

EVOLUTION OF PHYSICIAN COMPENSATION

The concept of integration between hospitals and physicians began to emerge in the 1980s and it has since taken on various structures and models. Today, we use the term alignment to describe these working relationships and how integration is reflected between physicians and hospitals. Over the last three decades, these arrangements have changed dramatically from their historical precursors. Some have resulted in engagement of physicians through "employment lite" models, such as a professional services agreement (PSA), as an alternative to full employment. With PSAs, these arrangements design compensation plans built upon a structure that aims to align incentives and overall goals and objectives of the physicians and the hospital. Figure 1.1.1 illustrates the movement of physician compensation plans.

In this overview, we will investigate first generation compensation plans—physician compensation plans in place over the last 30 years. We will also discuss their components, structures, and outcomes.

During the 1990s and earlier, incentives tied to productivity were few and far between. Due to this structure that lacks productivity tied to compensation, guaranteed compensation amounts were high. Additionally, significant benefits packages comprised a lucrative component of compensation as opposed to now, when a stronger focus is placed on productivity and benefits packages which, while still good, are not as rewarding as before. Minimal incentives or "stretch goals" were required of the physicians, the first indication that compensa-

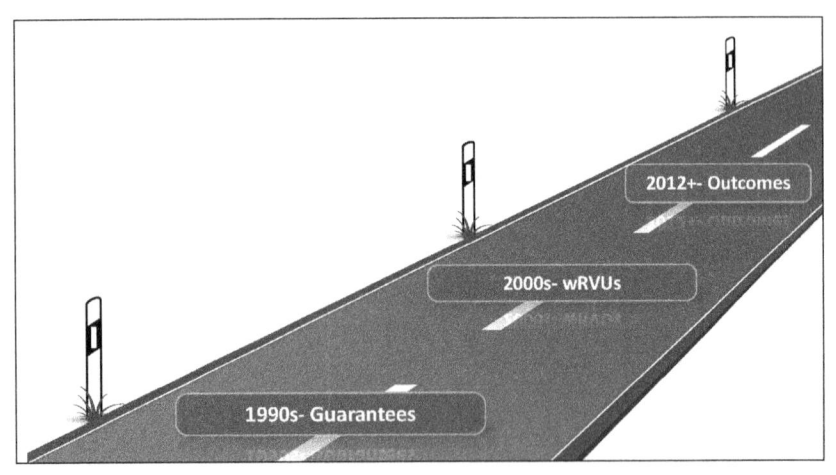

FIGURE 1.1.1 Movement of Physician Compensation Plans

tion plans based on guarantees were flawed. In the following years, it became apparent that due to the lack of incentives, achieving aligned goals between hospital and physicians would not likely be realized.

Productivity incentive became a stronger focus in the early 2000s with the emergence of work relative value units (wRVUs). Even so, most of the total compensation was tied to guarantees, and the percentage of incentive compensation remained low. Performance outside of productivity, too, remained limited in this decade. Performance incentives that would become pertinent to later compensation plans were not yet fully realized and implemented. Benefits during this time continued to be reasonable, but pensions were not off the table as an option. Guaranteed compensation was also largely dependent on the locality in which the physician practiced. Today, it is not uncommon to see physician incentives for practicing in rural locations, and conversely, increased compensation in higher-paying areas.

The 2010s saw an even stronger focus on productivity tied to compensation. New compensation plans began significantly emphasizing the inclusion of performance incentives in addition to productivity incentives that physicians aimed to reach. Subsequently, guarantees in compensation plans started decreasing as productivity and performance incentives increased. Benefits packages continued to remain reasonable, and the precedence of removing pensions in the 2000s endured. As we move into the second generation of physician compensation models, there are still uncertainties about how the healthcare landscape is chang-

1990s	• High guarantees • No productivity expectations • Significant benefit packages
2000s	• Strong focus on productivity (mainly wRVUs) • Guarantee treatment largely depends on locale • Limited performance incentives (outside of productivity) • Reasonable benefit package (no more pensions)
2010s	• Continued focus on productivity, although changing • Significant focus on inclusion of performance incentives (outside of productivity) • Decreasing guarantees • Reasonable benefit package (no more pensions) • Questions of what the future looks like

FIGURE 1.1.2 Key Changes in Physician Compensation

ing and how hospital or practice leadership will adapt to the changes going forward with physician compensation arrangements.

These models are shifting from volume to value in response to individual reimbursement and bundled payments that must spread across groups of providers. Because of this shift, reimbursement models of the past will not be applicable in the future. The previous models based on high guarantees are no longer affordable and are coming to an end. Modern compensation structures that are flexible and adaptable to the uncertain future of the market are now emphasized heavily. Figure 1.1.2 illustrates the key changes in physician compensation.

What Works in First Generation Compensation Plans

Historically, the physician compensation plans in place worked, and they continue to work today while the healthcare landscape is in flux. Nevertheless, reimbursement paradigms are the primary reason these first generation plans are inherently flawed and require restructuring in the future. Under the shifting healthcare environment, reimbursement structures will be predicated on physician productivity and outcomes; thus, there is a need for revised physician compensation plans that reflect the second wave of physician employment.

First generation physician compensation plans comprised several components that work in the healthcare industry and are considered worthy of moving into second generation compensation plans. These include provider accountability, which was introduced by implementing provider incentives. The transition from high guarantees to predictive incentives has increased productivity among physicians. Another strong influence from the current models is the involvement of both hospital/practice leadership and physicians in developing these compensation models. The requirement of periodic assessment helped to revise compensation plans and design based on where the hospital/practice is economically and how to best align its goals with physicians. Toward the end of the period of first generation compensation plans, the matter of quality and other non-productivity-based incentives are being introduced, which is becoming a more considerable indicator of compensation.

Reasons for Inherently Flawed Compensation Plans

Flaws of first generation compensation plans are mainly due to the structure of the compensation and incentives placed with the physicians at the start of those arrangements. Here, we discuss the reasons for flawed compensation plans and their repercussions.

1. Work RVUs (wRVUs) are a valid and useful tool for measuring productivity and deriving compensation, yet they can create opportunities to be manipulated and overstated, rather than directly relating them to the "real world" of actual reimbursed dollars. The tendency for physicians to be aggressive in accumulating productivity units and maximizing assigned CPT codes and converting them to higher wRVU rates has implications for flaws in the wRVU structured compensation plans. While not an overt act of abuse of the system or violations of Medicare, it is a natural human tendency to be aggressive in maximizing compensation. With expiring contracts under high-guarantee wages, hospitals are now reconsidering the best ways in which to renew these contracts under a similar wRVU productivity basis.
2. A second reason compensation plans of the past are flawed is the expectation many health systems had of taking market share away from their competitors. This expectation enabled them to justify losses from their newly employed or contracted physicians. Relatively "easy" incentives rationalized the high levels of compensation, yet this assumption has become harder to validate years later as the transactions' second generation approaches. Methods of remedying this situation include reducing physician compensa-

tion or increasing productivity without commensurately increasing compensation.

3. Lack of cost controls and containment represents another flaw in historical compensation structures. It is important to note that overhead accounts for nearly 50 percent of total healthcare costs, leaving the remaining 50 percent to cover compensation and benefits. Rarely did any traditional compensation models tie incentives to cost controls and containment; thus, physicians did not seek to do so. Additionally, a focus on productivity creates a disincentive for physicians to control costs. In response to this realization, hospitals are updating compensation models to include significant incentives tied to cost controls and containment. While many physicians believe they have little to no control of overhead expenses, employers continue to emphasize this component. Physicians who maintain the responsibility of controlling costs do earn a profit from the reimbursement for those expenses they receive from the health system.

4. In addition to a lack of cost controls and containment incentives, historical compensation models lacked non-productivity-based incentives in areas that have become increasingly important relative to accountable care era structures and approaching changes in overall reimbursement. These factors, such as patient satisfaction, reaching quality metrics, and other non-productivity-based incentives, are becoming more relevant to the second generation structures. Physicians view these types of non-productivity measures as difficult to quantify and thus prefer wRVU and productivity-based structures. However, as the reimbursement paradigm changes, encompassing bundled payments and other similar types of reimbursements, it is vital to implement these types of non-productivity incentives.

5. Lastly, the lack of partnering mentalities from both the hospital leaders and the physicians has resulted in flawed compensation structures. A minimal discussion toward governance and joint partnership structures led to a lack of unity within the health system, resulting in misalignment of overall goals and objectives. More recently, this lack of unity has been recognized and remedied through more stringent and considerable time spent on issues at hand and day-to-day management and oversight between hospital leaders and physicians. Renewed contracts have thus detailed part-

nership efforts and units of governance to enhance a closer working relationship between the two parties.

Why Compensation Models Have Not Succeeded

First generation compensation models have not been successful for several reasons. Frequently, these issues are reaching a resolution in the second generation compensation plans. Second generation plans take into consideration the shift to the accountable care era, focusing on value rather than volume. It is not surprising that physicians are challenging these changes. Thus, it is important to articulate the reasons historical compensation models cannot continue in the same manner in light of the changing reimbursement paradigm. We will briefly provide an overview of the primary reasons the first generation compensation plans have been unsuccessful with more details to follow in later chapters.

The guarantee of too much base pay and the lack of incentives were apparent in previous contracts. In addition to affecting outcomes, lack of incentives affected physician behavior and was reflected in the lack of productivity, lack of cost control consciousness, lack of accountability for patient satisfaction, and inefficiency throughout the healthcare system.

In addition to high guaranteed base pay, "easy" incentives in first generation contracts were obvious. Having easily obtainable incentives can exacerbate the problem of excessive "earned" compensation. Conversely, incentives should not be so high that they are unattainable, which would be disincentives for physicians to produce at high levels.

When first generation compensation contracts were negotiated, many health systems had the mindset of formulating the pay structure now and worrying about its effects later. The lack of planning and failure to address tough issues early on has resulted in the closer scrutiny of new contracts. The reason for approving high base pay was to stabilize the provider base and/or increase the market share. As an aside to this, physicians were not always fully educated about the expectations of their employment and the overall performance measures. This lack of knowledge created an environment conducive to lapses in physician performance; thus, they are being corrected going forward.

As mentioned earlier, the lack of a true partnership between the hospital leaders and physicians did not encourage an environment of collaboration and cohesiveness. The lack of foresight regarding

Chapter 1—Overview of Compensation Plans

```
┌─────────────────────────────────────────────────────────────────┐
│              Traditional Healthcare Delivery Model              │
└─────────────────────────────────────────────────────────────────┘
```

Fragmented care management treating primarily sick people	Episodes of care; utilization management	Predominantly production (volume)/fee-for-service payments	Disjointed provider base
Integrated care management focusing on preventative care	Coordinated delivery of care rendering appropriate services at appropriate place and time	Performance (value); Quality/cost control; bundled payments; capitation; risk-based	Collaboratives: ACOs/CINs/PCMHs / QCs

```
┌─────────────────────────────────────────────────────────────────┐
│              Accountable Care Era Healthcare Delivery           │
└─────────────────────────────────────────────────────────────────┘
```

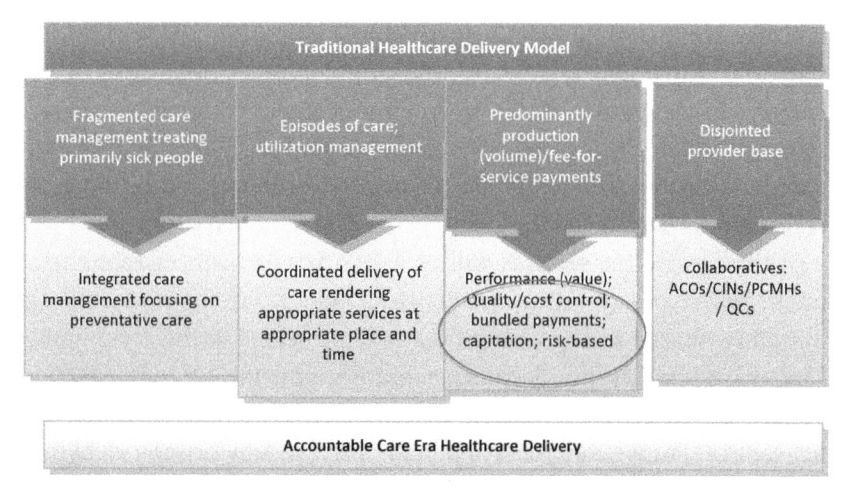

FIGURE 1.1.3 Traditional Healthcare Delivery Model

the ramifications and expectations of physician performance are now being met negatively by physicians going forward. Historic compensation plans did not emphasize the matter of collaboration, and hospitals now rely on tougher terms in their updated agreements.

Checks and balances between the health system and physicians ultimately determine the worth and overall effectiveness of an employment incentive contract. It is essential to incorporate checks and balances into a partnership for both parties to maintain their performance and overall behavior. Previously, few of these checks and balances between the parties were in place, and as such, the contracts under this structure have been unsuccessful. Figure 1.1.3 illustrates the transition of the traditional healthcare delivery model to the accountable care era of healthcare delivery.

Second Generation Compensation Plan Considerations (to be detailed in later chapters)

Second generation compensation plans present various matters and issues to address regarding mistakes made in first generation compensating plans. The overarching goal in developing second generation compensation plans is to address the necessity of the employer-employee working relationships. By making this concept a priority, all subsequent policies and actions should occur with this concept in mind. While creating a new and updated compensation plan is a massive undertaking, it is achievable if all parties involved understand the value and benefit of renewing contracts, regardless of the changes in compensation terms. In light of the impending reimbursement paradigm changes, physician and hospital alignment is critical for success. Here, we briefly discuss the market evolution and future goals considerations involved in second generation compensation plans.

Although fee-for-services will remain a major form of reimbursement, new types of reimbursement, including pay for performance, bundling, shared savings, etc., will come into effect in the accountable care era of healthcare. Second generation and future compensation plans must reflect these structures as standards, more so than just fee-for-service. Future compensation plans also must incorporate a hybrid of productivity- and non-productivity-based incentives. This change should be evident, but not drastic, in the total percentage of compensation tied to non-productivity-based incentives.

As noted above, fee-for-services will continue as the primary compensation driver, yet exclusive emphasis on productivity-based compensation will likely obstruct the ability to address other priorities. Other important factors to address include access and management of populations, integration of physician specialties, and other healthcare providers as a continuum of care, and raising the quality of clinical care. This structure facilitates increased awareness and incentive where group production/performance is necessary. Compensation in this arrangement may fall under bundled reimbursement structures tied to clinically integrated networks, where both the physician and hospital services are provided.

Go-Forward Solutions

Moving forward, collaboration must occur between hospital leaders and physicians to address the flaws of first generation compensation arrangements. As the healthcare market shifts into the accountable care era, newer, updated models must be implemented to address this shift to be responsive to both market and industry conditions that currently exist. As emphasized earlier, subtle, not drastic changes, will occur. This section will briefly provide an overview to some possible go-forward solutions to second generation compensation. (More details will be reviewed in later chapters.)

The primary reason compensation structures must change is the shift away from fee-for-volume to fee-for-value. This shift may require redefining or replacing productivity. Moreover, the addition of new incentive components tied to accountable care era methodologies should be enhanced.

Evolving incentives should be illustrated as an evolutionary process for implementing non-productivity-based incentives. In cases where the second generation contract is for an extended term, non-productivity incentives should be understood as part of the compensation components and likely will be phased in over time. Factors of non-productivity incentive should be tied to specific performance measures and cost control and containment.

CONCLUSION

Quality and efficiency measurements fluctuate, and, as such, it is necessary to consider them annually to tie performance to compensation appropriately. Through annual updates, these measures can be modified to respond to the needs of the healthcare system. These actions may include financial and clinical performance, improve patient care metrics, and drive patient and physician satisfaction metrics.

SECTION I

CHAPTER 2

Current First Generation Plans

HISTORY OF PHYSICIAN COMPENSATION MODELS

During the 1990s and earlier, compensation was mostly guaranteed with minimal incentives or "stretch goals" required of the physicians. As a result, guaranteed amounts were high and little money was tied to productivity. During this first wave of employment, compensation arrangements fell short in achieving aligned incentives due to the lack of a productivity requirement tied to compensation. Further, these early plans featured lucrative benefits packages with pension plans for most physicians. As a result, the compensation plans were desirable to physicians and costly to their employers.

A stronger focus was put on productivity in the early 21st Century to combat high guarantees, mostly tied to work relative value units (wRVUs). Much of the total compensation package, starting in 2000, was linked to some form of guaranteed income, and overall, the percentage of incentive compensation was low (i.e., the percentage of the total of incentives to total compensation). Due to large guaranteed salaries from years prior, the focus shifted to wRVU productivity wherein a portion of compensation was tied to exceeding an established wRVU threshold. Performance incentives were also introduced with a minimal amount tied to achieving metrics not measured by wRVUs. Benefits packages that were in these newer arrangements were good, although they were not as lucrative as those in contracts from earlier years and pensions were eliminated from the benefits package.

In 2010, the introduction of the Affordable Care Act (ACA) shifted the focus from predominantly wRVU productivity to the inclusion of performance incentives to focus on improved quality and clinical outcomes. The value of performance metrics is increasing as a shift continues to occur in the reimbursement paradigm for healthcare professionals. Compensation plans still use wRVUs as the basis of compensation; however, guaranteed base salaries have been eliminated for the majority of physicians in favor of a draw on total cash compensation (projected by the prior year's productivity) as their base salary. Today, guaranteed salaries for physicians are rare and usually occur in rural markets where patient volumes are low. Benefits packages continue to be streamlined as more health systems, hospitals, and providers fall under federal scrutiny.

Refer to Section I, Chapter 1, Figure 1.1.2, for an illustration of the evolution of physician compensation (page 3).

Under these first generation compensation plans, many health systems expected to take market share away from their competitors, enabling them to justify losses from their newly employed physicians. It is not difficult to justify higher levels of compensation through "easy" incentives when market share is the opportunity that has been afforded. While this action may well have been justified from a business standpoint in the original transaction, this position is more difficult to accept five to seven years later as that transaction's second generation approaches and the compensation model does not generate total cash compensation in alignment with productivity or performance. Boards of directors and other leaders of health systems are increasingly insistent on a significant reduction in the direct losses from employed or fully aligned, contracted physicians. The best way to achieve financial improvements is through reductions in physician compensation. Conversely, financial improvement can occur by increasing productivity without commensurately increasing compensation.

The following section addresses the second wave of employment and the key features of the compensation models in place for current first generation plans.

SECOND WAVE OF EMPLOYMENT

In the second wave of physician employment, health systems were smarter, offering less in terms of guaranteed pay and more compensation tied to incentives. At the time, there was a minimal focus on "value-based care" and, therefore, practically all of the incentives were tied to volume. The models used a variety of volume metrics, with the key metric being wRVUs. While wRVUs are a valid and useful tool to measure productivity and derive compensation, they do not relate directly to the "real world" of actual dollars reimbursed. Furthermore, many physicians have been able to manipulate the system by knowing wRVU values (one relative to the other) and maximizing their assigned CPT codes and converting to higher wRVU rates. This statement is not an assertion that physicians overtly abuse the system; however, it is a natural human tendency to be aggressive in both coding and the overall accumulation of productivity units (i.e., wRVUs) when incentivized to do so. This model worked (when properly developed) in that there was a strong alignment between what drove physician compensation and what drove revenue, which at that time was predominantly, if not exclusively, fee-for-service work. The result is that, as the compensation plans with a high guaranteed wage (at least in the early years of the contract) are expiring, hospitals are reconsidering whether it is best to renew the contracts on a similar basis (i.e., wRVU productivity criteria).

Earlier compensation models that are now expiring also lacked non-productivity, performance-based incentives. Performance incentives include patient satisfaction, attaining quality metrics, and clinical outcomes. These types of incentives have become increasingly important relative to accountable care era structures and impending changes in the overall reimbursement paradigm. Physicians view these factors as somewhat onerous because measurements of metrics for patient satisfaction, quality, and similar performance indicators are difficult, if not somewhat nebulous, to quantify. Physicians prefer to produce wRVUs and to be paid more as a result of greater production rather than being measured by these indicators. Nonetheless, as reimbursement structures start to change and with the move to bundled payments and other similar types of reimbursement, it is essential to implement incentives that are tied to something other than productivity (e.g., wRVUs, or some other measure).

The following sections address the key tenets of first generation plans and introduce the options under consideration for future models.

Treatment of Base Compensation

The treatment of base compensation has evolved over the years from a completely guaranteed salary to at-risk, tied to specific productivity and performance metrics. During the 80s and 90s, total cash compensation was predominantly guaranteed with no value-at-risk based on productivity or performance requirements. With no value tied to additional incentives, individual physician production was often low and did not support the guaranteed salary from a reimbursement standpoint. Health systems and hospitals were beginning to see larger losses tied to physician compensation. Today, guarantees exist mainly in rural markets where patient volumes are low and cannot support a productivity-based compensation model. For the same reason, health systems and hospitals that have "mission-based" specialties (specialties and services necessary to fulfill a community need) will offer guaranteed salaries to physicians, although these are more commonly seen as a guaranteed base salary with the opportunity to earn additional incentive compensation.

As the salary approach started to phase out at the beginning of the 21st Century, many health systems and hospitals adopted a "base plus" approach where physicians were provided with a lower guaranteed base salary with the opportunity to earn additional incentive compensation based on wRVU productivity and certain quality-based initiatives. The base plus approach better aligned total cash compensation with productivity and incentivized physicians to increase their patient volumes. A minimal performance incentive, usually around $10,000, was tied to general quality and non-production-based metrics. Many of these were easily achievable and quickly became another add-on to compensation with little risk to the physicians. Today, these models are still fairly common for mission-based specialties and for compensating advance practice providers.

The introduction of the ACA in 2010 again shifted the focus of at-risk compensation from predominantly productivity to quality-based performance incentives. Treatment of base compensation also shifted from guaranteed status to a draw on total cash compensation. In many ways, this move may be directly related to the significant increase in federal scrutiny within the last two to five years. Health systems, hospitals, and physicians have been involved in a rash of lawsuits under the false claims and anti-kickback statutes related to the type and level of compensation physicians receive. As a result, compensation models are being redesigned to improve the alignment of total cash compensation with productivity and performance indicators, including treating base compensation as a draw on total cash compensation. Incentive compensation is only paid after the full value of base compensation has been earned under the compensation model. These plans also trigger an evaluation of the level of base compensation at the end of each contract year based on the physician's performance during that year.

As physician compensation, and the healthcare industry in general, are highly regulated, it is important to develop a compensation model that promotes compliance. The alignment of base compensation with the model drivers (primarily wRVU productivity in these first generation plans) is essential to generating compensation within a fair market value (FMV). From a base compensation perspective, initially setting the base too high can inherently misalign compensation with productivity, and completely guaranteeing base compensation creates the same problem. If physicians' productivity levels cannot support the total cash compensation ultimately earned, the arrangement will not be within FMV limitations and leaves the health system or hospital vulnerable from a compliance standpoint. The use of wRVUs allows employers to measure the work effort of the physician accurately and compare physician production to industry survey data. Thus, wRVU-based models have become a standard within the healthcare industry and represent the majority of current first generation plans.

The wRVU Model

Several years ago, the focus of physician compensation models was almost entirely based on production. The production models, while all slightly different, have similar elements; the majority included the use of wRVUs in some manner. Even today, wRVUs are a significant element in most physician compensation arrangements. The reason for the continued use of wRVUs in physician compensation is wRVUs render a truer measure of actual physician productivity than other measures that exist (charges, collections, units, etc.) and wRVUs are directly correlated to physician work and are not affected by practice expense or malpractice expense. Further, wRVUs measure complexity or severity and take into account physicians' effort, stress, judgment required, etc. They are also considered to be "payer blind," meaning a physician receives the same credit for commercial and indigent patients, and wRVUs can be consistently applied to all healthcare providers. Lastly, wRVUs do not penalize a physician or skew data for operational inefficiencies, which is paramount in employed settings.

The wRVU model is also easy to manage with the same basic formula: wRVUs multiplied by the conversion factor equals total compensation. While the wRVUs are what they are, meaning they are driven by what the physician generates under the weighting established annually by an independent party, the conversion factor must be established. There is no set approach for deriving conversion factors and each health system approaches it differently; however, the most common approach is to use industry benchmark data.

Many key industry surveys provide physician compensation and productivity data. Three tend to be the most frequently used and the most universally accepted. These are the following:

- Medical Group Management Association (MGMA) Physician Compensation and Production Survey
- American Medical Group Association (AMGA) Medical Group Compensation and Financial Survey
- Sullivan, Cotter and Associates, Inc. (SCA) Physician Compensation and Productivity Survey

Each of these surveys is updated annually and provides a wealth of information on a variety of specialties and financial metrics, providing numerous different "slices" of the data. The key to establishing an appropriate conversion factor is to consider all elements of compensation (including non-productivity-based incentives) and determine a conversion factor around the median of industry data.

The structure of the wRVU model can range from a simple single-tier model to a multi-tiered model with varying conversion factors at each tier. Since their inception, wRVU models have increased in complexity (i.e., multiple tiers) to add depth to the model. A single-tier wRVU model establishes one conversion factor as the value of a single wRVU. Thus, on a productivity-only model, total compensation is equal to total wRVUs times the conversion factor.

Figure 1.2.1 is an illustration of a single-tier wRVU model where base compensation is paid at the single-tier conversion factor and treated as a draw on total cash compensation.

Single-Tier Model	Amount
Base Compensation	$125,000
wRVU Threshold	4,000
Conversion Factor	$31.25
wRVUs Produced	4,500
wRVU Compensation	$15,625
Total Compensation	$140,625[1]

FIGURE 1.2.1 Single-Tier wRVU Model

A multi-tier wRVU model establishes more than one conversion factor with which to pay physicians once certain wRVU thresholds are achieved. More often than not, we have found the added complexity to the model has more impact at a psychological level than an economic one. Further, as performance incentives continue to evolve, the added complexity of the productivity component becomes unwieldy to manage. As illustrated in Figure 1.2.2, the five-tier wRVU model adds significant complexity to the calculation of the model. As an example, if a physician produces 4,500 wRVUs on the five-tier model, 0 to 3,500 wRVUs are paid at a rate of $31.00 per wRVU, productivity exceeding 3,500 wRVUs up to 4,200 wRVUs are paid at a rate of $33.00, and productivity exceeding 4,200 wRVUs (in this case 300 wRVUs) are paid at a rate of $35.00.[2]

Tier	From	To	Incremental	Rate
I	0	3,500	3,500	$31.00
II	3,500	4,200	700	$33.00
III	4,200	4,900	700	$35.00
IV	4,900	5,600	700	$37.00
V	5,600			$40.00

FIGURE 1.2.2 Five-Tier wRVU Model

In the last few years, the introduction of at-risk performance incentives has added more complexity to these models such that we are starting to see less-complex wRVU-based components. However, many of these first generation plans treat performance incentives as an add-on to the compensation model with a small to moderate dollar amount tied to general, more easily achievable goals. The initial performance incentives, in many cases, were designed to garner physician buy-in to the model with the goal of integrating performance incentives more heavily into the model as the reimbursement paradigm began to shift.

Distributable Net Income (DNI) Model

The DNI model is another option under first generation plans and is also known as the private practice model, as it is seldom used in an employed setting. Historically, the "revenue-less-expense" model has always existed in private practice, wherein the revenue generated by a practice less the expenses incurred dictates the pool of compensation available for distribution to the respective physicians. This model works well when revenue is high and expenses are low, but when that is not the case, the model breaks down, as it no longer provides a market wage to the physicians. The less-than-market wage has been the case in recent years. Financial pressure on many private practices has forced them to give up their independence and to become employees of a health system so the health system can manage their practice and pay the physicians a market-based wage.

The upside to the DNI model is it inherently accounts for all sources of revenue, not just fee-for-service as with the wRVU model. Total cash compensation is equivalent to all revenue less all expenses under this model. It is more challenging under the wRVU model to account for sources of revenue other than fee-for-service and incentivize physicians to achieve performance targets for non-productivity-based metrics.

For healthcare providers, sources of revenue typically include the following:
- **Professional Fees (Fee-for-Service).** Reimbursement for all professional services the physician performs from commercial and government payers. Fee-for-service is the most prominent form of reimbursement for physician services under first generation contracts. Fundamentally, the fee-for-service reimbursement process simply means that providers of healthcare services receive a set fee for each unit of service they provide to patients.
- **Accountable Care Organization (ACO) Income.** After the introduction of the ACA, there has been a push to form ACOs to coordinate high-quality healthcare to Medicare patients. Through the reduction of costs and a focus on high quality clinical care, some organizations are receiving a second revenue stream for shared savings.
- **Third-Party Payer Initiatives:** Similar to the goals of an ACO, many third-party commercial payers are establishing a separate

fee schedule for non-productivity-based metrics. While fewer first generation contracts have these initiatives as a revenue source, it is becoming more prevalent within the healthcare industry. Under a wRVU model, these performance metrics are harder to integrate in the model to incentivize physicians to generate this type of revenue.
- **Capitation Fees.** Capitation fees, seen mostly in private practice settings, are paid to the practice or organization at a fixed amount, often on a per-patient basis, for the full management of that group of patients for a set period. The goal is to keep the total cost of the patient under or even within the amount paid to the organization. In the 1980s, as a combatant to the fee-for-service model, capitation arrangements began to see increasing prominence and while in existence today, capitation remains the least common source of revenue for healthcare providers.
- **Call Coverage.** Many private practice physicians receive call coverage payments from the hospitals for which they provide unassigned call. While less common in the employed setting, employed physicians can also receive additional compensation for call, typically in excess of an established baseline level.

Overhead expenses fall into four major categories: direct expenses, indirect expenses, physician base salary, and physician benefits. The details of each category are outlined below.
- **Direct Expenses.** A cost that is directly attributable to a service being offered, such as the physician, service-specific support staff, equipment, or supplies. While a direct expense, the physician cost is generally considered separately from all other direct expenses.
- **Indirect Expenses.** A cost that is attributable to maintaining the entire organization, such as general support staff and administration, insurance, rent, taxes, utilities, or office equipment.
- **Physician Base Salary.** The value of the draw on total cash compensation for the physician from all sources.
- **Physician Benefits.** The value of fringe benefits such as the employer's share of FICA, payroll and unemployment taxes, health, disability, life, and workers' compensation insurance, dues and memberships to professional organizations, professional development, state and local license fees, and employer payment

to defined benefits and contribution, 401(k), 403(b), and unqualified retirement plans.

The DNI model clearly identifies all revenue sources and all expenses with the remaining profit distributed among all physicians; however, as previously noted, this model breaks down if no profit is available. Within the last decade, healthcare expenses have steadily increased while reimbursement has decreased, leading to lower levels of compensation under this model. As it is essentially a private practice model, more physicians have opted for employment or another form of alignment to stabilize compensation. For the same reasons, health systems and hospitals use industry survey market data to determine appropriate levels of compensation under a wRVU model.

Future Models

So, why would the industry want to change the current structures? The answer is that issues with the compensation plans are becoming evident, and while physicians may be reasonably happy with their pay, their hospital employers are finding the models unsustainable. Reimbursement models of the past will not apply in the future. There is a significant shift from volume to value, from individual reimbursement to bundled payments, which must be spread across a group of providers. Further, many of the details of how this will play out in the marketplace are still unknown. Therefore, compensation structures of the past three decades are unaffordable, so they must come to an end. They must be replaced with models that are based on a shift from volume to value, and they must be flexible to allow for adaptation as the changes unfold.

CONCLUSION

The healthcare industry continues to shift from volume to value, and in doing so, has created the need to revise compensation plans across the board. The current first generation plans focus heavily on productivity and assume reimbursement based on a fee-for-service model. Since 2010, fee-for-value has continued to gather steam in the marketplace and many health systems, hospitals, and practices are being reimbursed for achieving value-based measures in addition to fee-for-service.

As fee-for-value continues to increase and displace fee-for-service, healthcare organizations need to adapt the compensation mechanism for physicians to balance volume and value. The key to updating first generation plans is to achieve this balance and incentivize physicians to achieve both productivity-based and performance-based metrics.

REFERENCES

1. 4,500 wRVUs x $31.25 = $140,625
2. Tier I: 3,500 wRVUs × $31.00 = $108,500
   Tier II: 700 wRVUs × $33.00 = $23,100
   Tier III: 300 wRVUs × $35.00 = $10,500
   Total: $108,500 + $23,100 + $10,500 = $142,100

SECTION 1

CHAPTER 3

Market and Industry Dynamics Promoting New Compensation Paradigms

The United States is recognized as one of the most expensive healthcare systems in the world. Health spending is measured by the increase in the nation's gross domestic product (GDP). From 1960 to 2013, the nation's healthcare spending rose from 5.0% of the GDP to 17.4%.[1] "After adjusting for economy-wide inflation (using the GDP price index), average annual growth was 5.5% between 1960 and 2013 compared to 3.1% growth in GDP."[2] As these data show, healthcare spending in the U.S. has increased almost twice as much as economic growth. Many estimate that by 2025, healthcare spending will reach an astronomical $5.631 trillion.

When comparing the per-capita costs of healthcare with other countries within the Organization of Economically Developed Countries (OECD), the United States leads in spending and in fact, in 2013 the United States spent approximately 50% more per capita on healthcare than the second most-expensive country, Switzerland ($9,086 versus $6,325), with the average cost per OECD country being $3,661.[2]

Both cost and non-cost factors are responsible for the growth in healthcare expenditures. In the 1960s and 1970s, the rise in costs was due primarily to the passage of Medicare and Medicaid.[1] As more people had access to health insurance, the usage of healthcare services, and as a result, costs, increased. The rise in healthcare costs in the 1970s and 80s was attributed to price inflation.[1] However, the reasons for the higher costs in the 1990s and 2000s were the result of the advent of managed care plans, as the nature of managed care plans shifted healthcare delivery from inpatient settings to outpatient settings, thus allowing more people to seek healthcare services.

Under the fee-for-service reimbursement model, payers based payment on medical necessity and whether or not a provider performed a service, and because there was no correlation between the value of the service and the amount the physician received as compensation, there was a strong incentive for the providers to increase the prices for said services.[3] As a result, the fee-for-service reimbursement system significantly contributed to the United States greatly outpacing the rest of the world in healthcare expenditures.[4] Further, this increased spending did not increase the quality of healthcare services provided in the United States compared to other industrialized countries.

When analyzing the quality of healthcare services, the United States ranks lower than the United Kingdom, France, and Germany.[5] High prices and lack of universal coverage led to the decrease in quality of services provided in the United States.[5] "A recent comparison of factors underlying differences in mortality rates from the leading amenable causes of death in the United States and the United Kingdom showed that many Americans failed to obtain recommended treatment for common chronic conditions and to secure regular, *affordable* treatment (emphasis added)."[5]

Studies have shown that a substantial number of deaths in the provision of healthcare can be prevented. While the definition of preventable harm is not universally agreed upon, we will assume that preventable harm is "unintended physical injury resulting from or contributed to by medical care (including the absence of indicated medical treatment), that require additional monitoring, treatment or hospitalization, or that results in death."[6] The most common types of preventable harm are hospital-acquired infections, performing surgery on the wrong site (e.g., the left arm instead of the right arm), medication errors, in-hospital injury (slip and falls), misdiagnosis, and deep vein thrombosis.[6]

In 1999, an estimated 99,000 patients died from preventable harm events in U.S. hospitals, and in 2014, this number increased to a staggering 400,000. Today, it is estimated that approximately 1,000 patients per day die as a result of preventable errors by providers. While these deaths lower the confidence patients have in their healthcare providers, a 2012 study demonstrated that these deaths also resulted in approximately $17 billion in additional medical bills and nearly $1.1 billion in lost productivity. If one includes indirect costs, the impact of preventable deaths could be as much as $1 trillion annually.[6]

Because not only did the increase in healthcare costs present an enormous burden on the U.S. economy but also did not lead to a similar increase in the quality of healthcare services, the U.S. government sought to fundamentally reform the way both healthcare services are monitored and also how providers are compensated for such services through the passage of the Patient Protection and Affordable Care Act of 2009 (ACA) and the Medicare Access and CHIP Reauthorization Act of 2015 (MACRA). In fact, the Secretary of the U.S. Department of Health and Human Services (HHS), who oversees the administration of Medicare through the Centers for Medicare and Medicaid Services (CMS), stated that HHS wants to have 30% of payments tied to alternative payment models, as permitted by MACRA (as explained below) by the end of 2016, and 50% by the end of 2018. HHS's second goal is to have 85% of payments tied to quality or value by the end of 2016, and 90% by the end of 2018.[7]

Dissatisfaction with Costs and Quality of Healthcare

As described above, healthcare costs are expected to increase through 2016 and beyond, with current projections stating that those costs will grow by 6.5% through 2017.[8] While this increase is less than what was seen before the passage of the ACA, the growth is still projected to outpace price inflation. Recognizing that the cost of healthcare is high, employers are taking a closer look at the value various health plans offer their employees. Specifically, companies are becoming increasingly dissatisfied with the payer's strategies for reducing waste and managing the overall health of the workforce population, as businesses are finding that payers are only providing for payment to treat an illness as opposed to overseeing the overall well-being of the patient.[9]

A result of this continual increase in healthcare costs is that many employers are shifting the costs to their workers by only offering high-deductible health plans, wherein the workers will need to shoulder the healthcare costs until their high deductible is met. It is estimated that 25% of employers currently offer a high-deductible plan, while another 39% of employers are considering a switch to such plans.[8] Additionally, many organizations are considering altering their health plans to that of a defined contribution plan, wherein an amount of money is set aside to pay for an employee's healthcare costs. After the employee's costs exceed the set-aside amount, the employee is responsible for the remainder of his or her costs for the rest of the year. Consequently, the number of employees who are satisfied with their employer-sponsored plans decreased from 69% in 2007 to 59% in 2013.[10] As a result of having to shoulder more of the burden of healthcare costs, fewer employees are willing to enroll (and sacrifice parts of their take-home pay) in their employer's health plan.

Finally, the dissatisfaction among healthcare costs does not end with employers and individual consumers; many payers are finding that it is not economically worthwhile to participate in the ACA-run insurance exchanges, nor is it wise to offer consumers a broad range of provider choices for the consumers due to the skyrocketing healthcare costs. In August 2016, the third-largest insurance company in the United States, Aetna, announced that it would no longer participate in most of the state-run insurance exchanges, citing losses of $430 million.[11] Aetna is not alone in this decision, as Anthem announced "it is projecting single-digit losses on the individual plans it sells on the exchanges for 2016. Humana said it would dial back its participation in the exchanges from 15 states to 11. UnitedHealth Group plans to remain on three or fewer exchange markets. Cigna has said that it is losing money on the exchanges."[11] Not only are many payers reducing their presence on the insurance exchanges, payers are limiting choice and competition by reducing the size of their physician networks.

As a result of the increase in healthcare costs, many insurers are reducing the size of their provider networks. A recent study found that roughly 40% of plans available on the state-run insurance exchanges are classified as small or extra-small provider networks.[12] In Colorado, hospitals were organized by either low-priced or high-priced hospitals. Those that were considered high-priced (and any physician associated with said hospitals) were removed from an insurer's plan.[13] Other insurers offer tiered networks as opposed to reducing the size of the network; however, the effect is relatively similar as patients will pay more healthcare costs depending upon the tier in which the provider is located. Not only do narrower networks reduce competition, they also reduce the quality of the networks available, as the networks are designed based on the costs to the payer and not based on the quality of care provided by the network.[13]

Value-Based Payment Reforms

While also expanding health insurance coverage through the creation of state and federally run health insurance exchanges, the ACA alters how providers are paid by "testing new delivery models and spreading successful ones, encouraging the shift toward payment based on the value of care provided, and developing resources for system-wide improvement."[14] One such reform established by the ACA is the Medicare Shared Savings Program, which allows for value-based reimbursement to those providers who deliver healthcare services through an ACO.

Value-based reimbursement for ACOs differs from a purely volume-based reimbursement model in that the ACO receives greater compensation if it achieves cost savings below predetermined levels set by CMS. In other words, CMS financially rewards ACOs for reducing the cost of treatment. Specifically, the ACO will be able to keep one-half of any achieved cost savings as compared with CMS-established cost benchmarks, with the other half of the savings being retained by CMS.[14] Along with the creation of ACOs, the ACA reduces annual rate increases in the Medicare Physician Fee Schedule, and the ACA mandates that CMS implement several reimbursement pilot programs such as the Bundled Care Payment Initiative.

The ACA mandated the initiation of various pilot projects that test alternative payments systems such as the implementation of bundled payments. One pilot project governed by CMS is the Bundled Care Payment Initiative (BCPI). The BCPI currently offers four tracks for the provider to receive bundled payments. "One model focuses on care provided during the hospital stay, while the other three models include post-acute care provided once the hospital discharges the patient."[15] CMS hopes that like other forms of value-based payments, the bundled payments will incentivize providers to coordinate with one another to provide more value to the patient receiving care instead of focusing on the number of procedures performed during a patient's course of treatment.[15]

MACRA enjoyed broad support among both political parties in Congress, and President Obama signed it into law on April 16, 2015.[16] MACRA introduced many payment reforms, including the elimination of the Sustainable Growth Rate (SGR) formula, which avoided a 21.2% cut in the Medicare Physician Fee Schedule.[16,17] MACRA also slows the Medicare Physician Fee Schedule's annual increases under the following schedule: annual increases by 0.5% from July 2015-2019; no increases after that until 2025; 0.75% annual increases for advanced Alternative Payment Model (APM) participants.[17] MACRA established the Medicare Incentive Payment System (MIPS) and the APM payment incentives. The APM participants and MIPS participants receive 0.25% annual increases for each year after 2025.[16] As stated earlier, along with slowing annual increases to the Medicare Physician Fee Schedule, MACRA established, as detailed *infra*, the MIPS, and APM payment incentives.

MACRA[7] established MIPS, which scores providers on various quality and cost-based categories. MIPS provides for payment adjustments to physicians' Medicare Part B payments, either by awarding bonuses or by requiring providers to remit payment to CMS, depending on how each provider compares to his or her peers in providing value to his or her patients.[7] "Performance and 'composite scores' under MIPS will be based upon four categories: quality (50 percent); resource use (10 percent); meaningful use (25 percent); and clinical practice improvement activities (15 percent)."[7] For those providers that score well against their peers, CMS will award up to a 4% payment increase in 2019, and up to a 9% payment increase in their Medicare Part B payments in 2022.[7] Because these payments must be budget-neutral, underperforming providers will be subject to a 4% reduction in 2019, and up to a 9% reduction in their Medicare Part B payments in 2022.[7]

For providers participating in certain demonstration and pilot programs administered by CMS or otherwise authorized by federal law, MACRA allows for reimbursement other than what is provided by MIPS. Specifically, providers who participate in the "SMC Innovation Center Model, the Medicare Shared Savings Program, any demonstration under the Health Care Quality Demonstration Program or otherwise authorized by federal law" will qualify as an APM.[7] Most of the providers that participate in APMs will still need to report data to the MIPS program, but those participants will receive only favorable adjustments to their clinical practice improvement activity scores, which accounts for 15% of their overall MIPS scores.[7] Select providers will qualify as advanced APM participants.

To qualify as a participant in an advanced APM, the entity must meet several requirements. First, to qualify as a participant in an advanced Alternative Payment Model, at least 50% of the eligible clinicians in each APM must use certified electronic health record technology to document and communicate clinical care. After the first year of participation, this requirement will increase to 75%. Second, the entity must base payments on quality measures comparable to those in the MIPS quality performance category. The entity must have at least one outcome measure unless there are no appropriate outcome measures available. Finally, the entity must bear risk for monetary losses, and that risk must meet a certain threshold, such as 4% of total expenditures and 30% marginal risk. Furthermore, the financial risk criteria for APMs require that if actual expenditures exceed expedited expenditures, there must be a direct payment from the APM to CMS or a reduction in payment rates the APM entity or eligible clinicians or withholding of payment to the APM or eligible clinicians.

CMS expects the following models to qualify as advanced APMs in 2017: (1) Medicare Shared Savings Plans (tracks 2 and 3); (2) Next Generation ACO Models; (3) Comprehensive End-Stage Renal Disease Care Models; and (4) Comprehensive Primary Care Plus and the Oncology Care Model (two-sided risk track available in 2018). Advanced APM participants will be given a 5% payment bonus annually, and will not be required to participate in MIPS reporting.[7] Those who are designated as having participated in non-advanced APMs will still be subject to the MIPS reporting requirements; however, those entities will not be subject to negative payment adjustments. Those providers who participate in advanced APMs will also receive higher annual increases in their Medicare Physician Fee Schedule as compared with those that do not qualify as advanced APM participants.[7]

While the government is seeking to factor in value to physicians' reimbursement, it is important to examine the operational transformation that providers will need to undergo to take advantage of the payment reforms instituted by the ACA and MACRA.

As is often the case, commercial insurance payers are following the lead of CMS and instituting value-based plans of their own. For example, EmblemHealth "has more than 60% of the HMO health plan members obtaining clinical services through a value-based care reimbursement arrangement," with the hopes of only increasing this percentage over time.[18] It is estimated that New York will have approximately 80% of its payments be value-based.

The numbers are even more staggering with UnitedHealthcare's plans: roughly $24 billion was awarded through the achievement of specific quality-based metrics, $2.5 billion was allocated to bundled payment initiatives that treat a particular condition or have a single service lines, and approximately $15 billion was awarded through population health and accountable care programs.[19]

Value-Based Payment Reforms Encourage Alignment and Clinical Integration

The value-based payment reforms instituted by the ACA and MACRA require many providers to align with one another in hopes of providing more value to their patients. To begin the transformation from fee-for-service reimbursement to value-based reimbursement, the method of healthcare delivery must change. One way to begin this transformation is for providers to form Integrated Practice Units (IPU) around specific conditions or CINs, which treat a large number of conditions.[20] While the members of the networks may be located in many geographical locations and while the providers may specialize in many different areas of care, the members of the IPUs or CINs work as a team to treat the patient's condition.[20] For example, data has shown that an IPU that treats back pain has resulted in its patients missing four fewer days of work and requiring four fewer physical therapy visits.[20] IPUs and CINs can involve primary care providers, with the emphasis here being on primary or preventive care for populations of patients, or specialist providers, with the emphasis here being on coordination of care around specific clinical conditions.

As stated earlier, to ensure that providers are providing value in the provision of their care, it is vital to be able to track healthcare outcomes. Practices that aren't integrated often do not have the ability to measure quality; their measurements instead center on legal compliance and practice guidelines.[20] However, to measure quality, the measurements should fall into three tiers. Tier one measures a patient's achieved health status—not just mortality rates but also activities patients can perform through the different stages of their recovery.[21] Measurements in the second tier relate to the patient's care cycle and recovery.[21] These measures include emergency room readmissions, the amount of pain experienced during the recovery process, and when a patient can resume regular activities.[21] The last tier of criteria relates to how long a person can expect to remain healthy or whether he or she will need subsequent procedures to maintain an ideal level of functionality.[21] These tiers cannot adequately be measured if a provider acts as a standalone entity; rather, many providers must work as a team to have access to the type of information necessary to adequately measure value.

Next, a provider must be able to properly measure costs relative to the treatment of the patient's underlying condition.[20] Many providers struggle with being able to measure costs relative to conditions, since most hospital accounting systems are based on a particular department and not on a patient's full cycle of care.[20] Further, most patient record systems measure charges and not the resources used to provide a full cycle of care for each patient.[20] Current patient record systems prevalent in small medical practices focus on the payments incurred for a particular procedure and are thus problematic in a value-based reimbursement environment since fee-for-service payments are continually decreasing.[20]

One possibility is for providers to transition to a time-driven activity-based costing system.[21] Time-driven activity-based costing involves "managers directly estimat[ing] the resource demands imposed by each transaction, product, or customer rather than to assign resource costs first to activities and then to products or customers."[22] This requires two measurements: "the cost per time unit of supplying resource capacity and the unit times of consumption of resource capacity by products, services, and customers."[22] Not knowing the amount of resources used when providing care for an underlying condition prevents an accurate determination of the amount of value the patient receives during their course of treatment.

Another important step in the transition from fee-for-service reimbursement to value-based reimbursement is integrating care among a multitude of providers.[20] Integrated systems must accomplish four tasks: "define the scope of services, concentrate volume in fewer locations, choose the right location for each service line, and integrate care for patients across numerous provider sites."[20]

Many provider networks do not integrate their care with other providers; rather, the providers in these networks operate as standalone providers that offer many of the same services in different locations.[20] Providing the maximum amount of value requires integrated networks to eliminate or narrow the scope of services that networks provide their patients, as the offering of multiple service lines typically results in an inefficient use of resources when providing treatment to the patient.[20] Further, it is important for networks to decide which conditions they want to treat. "Providers with significant experience in treating a given condition have better outcomes along with a reduction in costs."[20] When a network removes service lines that are duplicated across multiple locations, the network increases the volume of the relevant cases to a few locations.[20] To integrate care, it is important for the central entity to coordinate the patient's care across multiple network sites.[20] "Integrating mechanisms, such as assigning a single physician team captain or nurse navigator for each patient and adopting standard scheduling and other protocols, help ensure that well-coordinated multidisciplinary care is delivered in a cost-effective and convenient way."[20]

Besides forming and executing the integration plan, one of the most formidable obstacles in transitioning to value-based reimbursement is obtaining the necessary IT processes. Most IT systems in small practices, assuming the practice has an IT system, concentrate data by "department, location, type of service, and type of data."[20] However, to adequately capture value, the IT system must have many components.

First, the system must have the data centered on the patient.[20] The IT system also must be able to capture varying types of information, including "physician notes, images, chemotherapy orders, lab tests, and other data that is stored in a single place" so that all providers across different locations can have access to the necessary information when providing care to the patient.[20] The system should have templates that allow for easy entry of the data.[20] These information systems identify the processes of care for that condition as well as identify risks the patient will encounter during treatment.[20] Finally, the system must allow for an easy extraction of the data.[20] As healthcare transitions from a volume-based reimbursement model to a value-based model, it will be necessary for smaller practices to form and execute an alignment strategy that best fits that clinician's goals and needs.

Alternative Methods to Reduce Costs and Increase Quality

This rise in health costs has affected not only the individual consumer but also large employers that administer self-funded plans. These organizations have found that one way to reduce costs while ensuring high-quality of care is to contract directly with providers for the treatment of individual networks or certain conditions. For example, Wal-Mart has contracted with the Cleveland Clinic for certain cardiac and spine surgical procedures, while Boeing contracts with two ACO groups.[23,24]

Contracting directly with individual providers aids employers in multiple areas. First, the employer can expect to pay a certain price for every procedure, as opposed to paying different prices according to where the employee is treated. Second, these direct-contracting arrangements allow for the employers to contract for bundled payments instead of paying a separate fee for a number of different procedures that are related to one underlying condition (such as a knee or hip replacement). This not only reduces the costs of healthcare but also improves the quality of services, as Geisinger Health System "has seen a 21 percent reduction in complications, a 25 percent reduction in surgical infections and a 44 percent drop in readmissions."[24] Such programs also aid a health system, as contracting with a large employer such as Boeing or Intel provides the health system with a large patient base.[25]

Along with employers directly contracting with individual providers for healthcare services, some providers are finding additional ways to reduce costs, increase quality, and differentiate themselves from other healthcare providers by offering patients warranties for certain procedures. Geisinger Health System first offered warranties for surgical procedures,[26] whose warranty states that if the patient encounters any problems or complications within the first 90 days, any remaining costs for the patient's treatment are not charged to the patient.[26] The warranty offered by Geisinger Health System for total hip replacement surgery includes complications such as a hip dislocation or a blood clot in the leg; problems with the implant are not covered since that issue would need to be addressed with the implant manufacturer.[26]

However, this arrangement remains uncommon, and warranties are typically offered only for joint replacement surgeries, spine surgery, and open heart surgery, as the treatment plan and patient progression through the treatment plan are somewhat predictable. Further, the warranty program is mostly popular with self-insured employers and other self-paying patients such as medical tourists.[27] While the warranty program improves quality and reduces costs, many providers are concerned about offering such an option due to "the administrative burden, state regulatory uncertainty, and disagreements about bundle definition and assumption of risk."[27]

Need to Align Physician Compensation with Reimbursement Reforms

The transactions that have occurred over the past approximately five years have been flawed, mainly due to the structure of the compensation and incentive plans with the physicians at the outset of those agreements. Most of those contracts' incentives are based on a wRVU productivity plan. While wRVUs are a valid and useful tool to measure productivity and derive compensation, they do not relate directly to the "real world" of actual dollars reimbursed. Furthermore, many physicians have been able to manipulate the system by knowing RVU values (one relative to the other) and maximizing their assigned CPT codes and converting to higher RVU rates. This is not an assertion that physicians overtly abuse the system and commit violations of Medicare and other regulations. It is a natural human tendency to be aggressive in both coding and the overall accumulation of productivity units (i.e., wRVUs) when incentivized to do so. The result is that, as the compensation plans with a high guaranteed wage (at least in the early years of the contract) are expiring, hospitals are reconsidering whether it is best to renew the contracts under similar basis (i.e., wRVU productivity criteria).

Models have been flawed for many reasons, one of which is because they did not provide any significant incentives tied to cost controls. Overhead approximates 50% or more; the remaining 50% or more is dedicated to provider compensation and benefits. The compensation models that were established approximately five plus years ago under the new era of physician alignment/integration rarely included any significant incentives tied to costs and the control of overhead. Thus, because the employed/contract physicians had no incentive to control expenses, they have not done so. Further, in a highly-productivity-based incentive compensation model structure, there is a disincentive for the physician to control costs. Thus, as the new contracts are being consummated, health systems are offering an updated version that encompasses significant amounts of incentives tied to cost containment and control.

Physicians find this concerning, for many believe that they have very little to do with controlling overhead of a practice, particularly in an employed setting. Under updated models, the physicians maintain the responsibility of controlling costs and, in many instances, those who do a good job can realize a slight profit from the reimbursement for those expenses they receive from the health system. This factor makes PSA models very attractive and favorable, indicating they will continue to be so in the near- and longer-term future. For these reasons, it is important to ensure that physician compensation plans properly align with the various reimbursement and alignment reforms discussed in this and other chapters.

CONCLUSION

For several decades, the cost of healthcare has continued to rise, to the point that costs are substantially outpacing the growth of the economy, making it more unaffordable and inaccessible. As a result, the U.S. policymakers passed the ACA and MACRA, which incentivizes payers to produce a higher quality of healthcare for lower costs (i.e., value). To provide more value, providers are being required to integrate their care with other providers through the use of clinically integrated networks and accountable care organizations. This requires the new reimbursement models to be aligned with physician compensation models.

REFERENCES

1. Catlin A and Cowan C. History of health spending in the United States, 1960-2013. Centers for Medicare & Medicaid Services. November 19, 2016. https://www.cms.gov/Research-Statistics-Data-and-Systems/Statistics-Trends-and-Reports/NationalHealthExpendData/Downloads/HistoricalNHEPaper.pdf.
2. Squires D and Anderson C. U.S. health care from a global perspective. Commonwealth Fund. October 8, 2015. http://www.commonwealthfund.org/publications/issue-briefs/2015/oct/us-health-care-from-a-global-perspective.

3. State Health Care Cost Containment Commission. Cracking the code on health care costs: A report by the State Health Care Cost Containment Commission. University of Virginia Miller Center. 12. January 2014. http://web1.millercenter.org/commissions/healthcare/HealthcareCommission-Report.pdf.
4. Laugesen MJ and Glied, SA. Higher fees paid to U.S. physicians drive higher spending for physician services compared to other countries. *Health Aff 2011 Sep*;30(9):1647-1656. http://content.healthaffairs.org/content/30/9/1647.full.pdf+html.
5. Nolte E and McKee, CM. In amenable mortality—Deaths avoidable through health care—Progress in the US lags that of three European countries. *Health Aff.* 2012 Sep;31(9):2114-2122.
6. Newhook, E. What you should know about preventable harm. MHA@GW blog. Milken Institute School of Public Health, The George Washington University. August 31, 2015. https://mha.gwu.edu/blog-preventable-harm/. Accessed October 2, 2016.
7. CMS. *Medicare Access and CHIP Reauthorization Act of 2015 Path to Value. Centers for Medicare & Medicaid Services.* https://www.cms.gov/Medicare/Quality-Initiatives-Patient-Assessment-Instruments/Value-Based-Programs/MACRA-MIPS-and-APMs/MACRA-LAN-PPT.pdf. Accessed October 2, 2016.
8. Lorenzetti L. Here's why you'll likely pay more for your employer-sponsored health insurance. *Fortune.* June 21, 2016. http://fortune.com/2016/06/21/health-care-rising-costs. Accessed October 6, 2016.
9. Cantiupe J. More employers unhappy with health insurers, says PWC study. Media Health Leaders. January 19, 2010. http://www.healthleadersmedia.com/health-plans/more-employers-unhappy-health-insurers-says-pwc-study#. Accessed October 6, 2016.
10. Zane Benefits. Small business employee benefits and HR blog. Zane Benefits. May 12, 2014. https://www.zanebenefits.com/blog/employees-increasingly-unhappy-with-employer-sponsored-health-benefits-study. Accessed October 6, 2016.
11. Johnson C. Aetna will leave most Obamacare exchanges, projecting losses. Washington Post. August 16, 2016. https://www.washingtonpost.com/news/wonk/wp/2016/08/16/aetna-pulls-back-from-the-obamacare-exchanges/. Accessed October 6, 2016.
12. Ferris, S. Doctor networks shrinking under Obamacare, study finds. *The Hill.* June 24, 2015. http://thehill.com/policy/healthcare/246006-doctor-networks-shrinking-under-obamacare-study-finds. Accessed October 6, 2016.
13. Semro, B. Narrowing provider networks is all about cutting costs, but it also can lead to lower premiums. *Huffington Post.* October 3, 2014. http://www.huffingtonpost.com/bob-semro/narrowing-provider-networ_b_5928554.html. October 6, 2016.
14. *The Affordable Care Act's Payment and Delivery System Reforms: A Progress Report at Five Years.* The Commonwealth Fund. may 2015. http://www.commonwealthfund.org/publications/issue-briefs/2015/may/aca-payment-and-delivery-system-reforms-at-5-years. Accessed August 12, 2016.

15. Health Policy Brief: Bundled payments for care improvement initiative. *Health Aff.* 2015 Nov 23;1. http://healthaffairs.org/healthpolicybriefs/brief_pdfs/healthpolicybrief_148.pdf.
16. *Medicare Access and CHIP Reauthorization Act of 2015 (MACRA), H.R. 2, Pub. Law 114-10*. American Medical Association. May 7, 2015.
17. Cragun E. The most important details in the SGR repeal law. *Advisory Board*. April 20, 2015. https://www.advisory.com/research/health-care-advisory-board/blogs/at-the-helm/2015/04/sgr-repeal; Goldstein J. Why Medicare pay cuts for doctors will Be Back, *Wall Street J.*, (July 10, 2008), http://blogs.wsj.com/health/2008/07/10/why-medicare-pay-cuts-for-doctors-will-be-back/.
18. Gruessner V. Value-based care reimbursement makes strides in health plans. *Health Payer Intelligence*. February 22, 2016. http://healthpayerintelligence.com/news/value-based-care-reimbursement-makes-strides-in-health-plans. Accessed October 2, 2016.
19. UnitedHealthcare Services. *Customer's guide to self-funded value-based payment incentive programs*. United Healthcare Services. https://www.uhc.com/content/dam/uhcdotcom/en/NationalAccounts/PDFs/value-based-incentives-employer-guide.pdf. Accessed October 2, 2016.
20. Porter M and Lee T. The strategy that will fix health care. *Harvard Business Review*. October 2013. https://hbr.org/2013/10/the-strategy-that-will-fix-health-care.
21. Porter ME, and Tesiberg EO., *Redefining health care: creating value-based competition on results*. Boston: Harvard Business School Press; 2006.
22. Anderson S and Kaplan R. Time-driven activity-based costing. Harvard Business Review. November 2004. https://hbr.org/2004/11/time-driven-activity-based-costing.
23. Adamopoulos H. Working together to contain costs: What hospital leaders need to know for successful direct contracting with employers. *Becker's Hospital Rev*. June 27, 2014. http://www.beckershospitalreview.com/finance/working-together-to-contain-costs-what-hospital-leaders-need-to-know-for-successful-direct-contracting-with-employers.html. Accessed October 5, 2016.
24. Carabello L. Employer direct contracting: Game changing medical travel trend. Medical Travel Today. March 5, 2015. http://medicaltraveltoday.com/employer-direct-contracting-game-changing-medical-travel-trend. Accessed February 18, 2017.
25. Stempniak M. Will Boeing change health care? Hospitals & Health Networks. December 10, 2015. http://www.hhnmag.com/articles/6709-will-boeing-change-health-care. Accessed October 5, 2016.
26. Zamosky L. Considering surgery? Some healthcare providers offer warranties. *Los Angeles Times*. September 14, 2014. http://www.latimes.com/business/la-fi-healthcare-watch-20140914-story.html. Accessed October 6, 2016.
27. Le S. Warranties for medical procedures: Can they work? *Epoch Times*. September 24, 2014. http://www.theepochtimes.com/n3/976850-warranties-for-medical-procedures-can-they-work. Accessed October 6, 2016.

SECTION I

CHAPTER 4

"Second" Generation Compensation Models

INTRODUCTION

Why Compensation Models Matter

The importance of physician compensation arrangements cannot be understated because the structure of the compensation arrangement largely drives the behavior of the physician. It is akin to the rudder of a ship: turn it one way and the entire direction of the ship changes; turn it the other way and, again, the direction of the ship changes. Likewise, a physician group is similar to a massive ocean liner: it takes a lot to make the ship change course, but once it does, a lot of force is moving in a single direction.

Healthcare organizations have a set of goals and objectives for the future. Further, they often have established mission/vision/values that are driving the goals and objectives. The physician compensation arrangement should be aligned with such. As the goals and objectives of the organization change, the physician compensation arrangements should be updated accordingly. This adjustment is no small feat. As we discuss, below, many things are changing in the healthcare realm and, therefore, maintaining a compensation structure that is consistent with the market and the goals and objectives of the organization can be extremely challenging, especially when much of the future is unknown.

New Terms Introduced

A key to understanding and developing second generation compensation models is familiarity with some of the key terms that come into play. Below, we highlight and define the key terms that will play a role in the rest of the chapter. Some of this terminology may also be used elsewhere in the book and carry a similar definition/meaning.

- **Second Generation Compensation Model.** New models that include a more significant focus on factors outside of pure professional production. These models are not relegated to a particular period but typically were instituted after 2014.
- **First Generation Compensation Model.** Models that were put into place at the onset of employment arrangements over the last 5 to 10 years that were predominantly focused on professional production.
- **Productivity Incentives.** Still very common in second generation compensation models, this term includes wRVU-based or collections-based incentives tied to personal production.
- **Performance Incentives.** Incentives that are outside of professional production. The most common buckets include quality, patient satisfaction, and citizenship, but they can also include things such as expense control, coding and compliance, and other measures. All second generation compensation models include some form of performance incentives.
- **Scorecard.** The means of determining how much of the Performance Incentive a provider has earned. Typically, the score card looks something like the table below. As in the illustration (Figure 1.4.1), in certain models, the scorecard could also incorporate any productivity incentive.
- **Total Cash Compensation.** This term includes all forms of compensation that would typically show up on a provider's W-2, 1099, or K-1, including base compensation, production incentive, performance incentives, call pay, medical director pay, etc. It **does not** include benefits, such as employer-paid payroll taxes, health insurance, retirement plan contributions, etc. The definition of total cash compensation plays a role in market survey data as one of the key data points that they report.
- **External Incentives.** These incentives include new sources of revenue coming from external sources, such as ACOs, commercial payers, CINs, and others. The funds are typically tied to achievement of certain quality metrics, shared savings generated,

FIGURE 1.4.1 Scorecard

Incentive Compensation Matrix - Year Two				
Total Potential Incentive (Annual)			$45,000	
Components	Potential Points	Allocation	Potential $	Assigned Score
Productivity Incentive	50.0	50.00%	$22,500	20.0
Based on wRVUs above 4,000 baseline				
Scoring System				
Between 3,000 and 4,000 wRVUs	30.0			
Between 4,000 and 5,000 wRVUs	40.0			20.0
Greater than 5,000 wRVUs	50.0			
Performance Incentive	50.0	50.00%	$22,500	60.0
Quality, PULSE, Citizenship				
Scoring System				
Quality—below 75% on Quality Scorecard	20.0			20.0
Quality—above 75% on Quality Scorecard	30.0			
	5.0			20.0
Citizenship—below 75% on Citizenship Scorecard	10.0			
Citizenship—above 75% on Citizenship Scorecard	5.0			20.0
	10.0			
PULSE - below average on survey				
PULSE - above average on survey				
Totals	100.0	100.00%	$45,000	80.0
Total Points Earned			80.00	
Maximum Points			100.00	
Percentage of Incentive Earned			80.00%	
Total Incentive			$36,000	

or activities that a party sees as enhancing the health of a population. Sometimes these incentives are tied to specific providers, while other times their aggregation is at the medical group level. We expect these forms of revenue to increase in the future, in many cases replacing fee-for-service revenue.

- **Internally Funded Incentives.** In many (if not most) cases, the funding of performance incentives is through a reallocation of or in addition to current compensation dollars—meaning a healthcare provider simply designates some portion of compensation spend to focus on performance incentive metrics, regardless of whether they are generating additional revenue. Often, the metrics are seen as value-added regardless of their impact on revenue.

- **wRVUs.** The most common form of productivity measurement for physicians, wRVUs are based on the Resource-Based Relative Value Scale (RBRVS), which is used by Medicare and other payers to determine Part B reimbursement. For additional information on wRVUs, please reference Greenbranch Publishing's book titled *RVUs at Work: Relative Value Units in the Medical Practice, Second Edition*.
- **Panel.** Most commonly applicable to primary care, panel references the base of patients a particular physician is managing at any given time. The most common industry definition for patient panel is unique patients seen in the last 18 months. Alternatively, these data can be derived from the practice management system if the "primary care physician" field is maintained. For primary care, panel becomes important in second generation compensation models.
- **Top-Down Approach.** An approach to developing a compensation model wherein a certain level of overall economics is targeted, whether stated in the form of total cash compensation or total cash compensation per wRVU, and then the value is allocated to the various components of compensation in the model.
- **Market Survey Data.** Information pulled from market resources often used to establish the economics of a compensation arrangement. While many sources are available, industry-wide, the most common are Medical Group Management Association, American Medical Group Association, and Sullivan, Cotter, and Associates.

Challenge of Change

Change in any facet of life is never easy, and this is a major understatement on something as personal as provider compensation. In a stable environment, change is difficult, and in a rapidly evolving environment change is even harder to handle. This uncertainty is where the healthcare industry is today: lots of change, the feeling that provider compensation arrangements need to change, but limited knowledge as to how the future will truly look. There are glimpses, as we consider what is going on with MACRA, bundled payments, ACOs, etc., but even these new reimbursement schemes are immature and evolving.

Further, many providers perceive we are moving from something very black/white and objective (i.e., personal production) to something much grayer and subjective (i.e., performance incentives). Coupling this with the fact that more compensation is "at risk" relative to these unknown/evolving metrics and it is a recipe for many challenges (disaster is likely too negative of a word, but in many cases, it is not far from that).

Another key challenge of change is the composition of many healthcare organizations' medical groups. In most cases, the medical groups grew over time through acquisitions and the addition of physicians from outside the market. This scenario often resulted in rapid growth over a short period and a number of different compensation arrangements in place. Meaning, every physician in the organization is not on the same compensation framework. Thus, tweaking compensation arrangements is challenging, at best, in that there is no single platform to change. Either part of the modification must involve developing that single platform, or it will require tweaking/tampering with every single model structure that is in place. Managing the latter on a long-term basis, in the evolving market we are in, will continue to be problematic.

Hospital Employment

Over the last decade, the physician market has changed dramatically, with many physicians becoming employed by health systems. As was discussed in earlier chapters, this shift has had a dramatic effect on compensation strategies. What has been most notable about the change in compensation strategies as physicians have moved into hospital employment is that the focus is no longer solely on practice financial performance but relies on other measures of productivity. What is interesting about this shift is that a private practice model tends to work the best in a changing reimbursement environment. Figure 1.4.2 is an illustration of a private practice model profit and loss statement.

Prior to value-based reimbursement, it was a rather simple calculation. Professional fee revenue less direct expenses equaled physician compensation. With new forms of revenue, the calculation becomes a bit more complicated, but it still follows the same pattern. That is, revenue less expenses equals physician compensation. What is nice about this approach is that the model structure accepts all forms

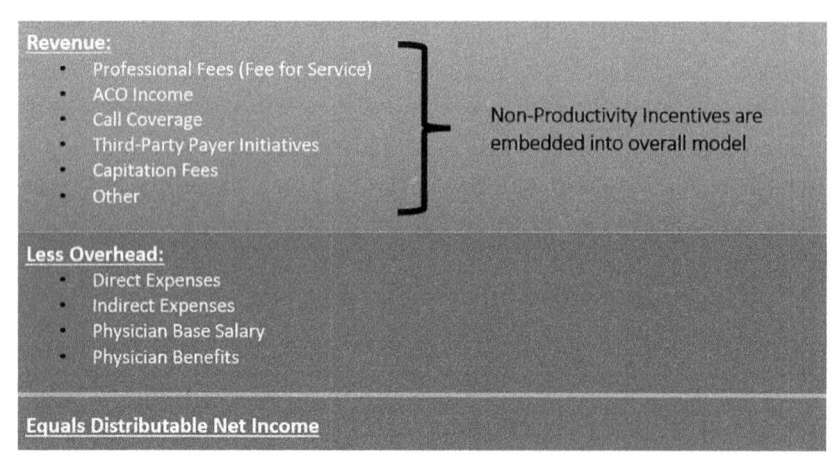

Revenue:
- Professional Fees (Fee for Service)
- ACO Income
- Call Coverage
- Third-Party Payer Initiatives
- Capitation Fees
- Other

} Non-Productivity Incentives are embedded into overall model

Less Overhead:
- Direct Expenses
- Indirect Expenses
- Physician Base Salary
- Physician Benefits

Equals Distributable Net Income

FIGURE 1.4.2 Private Practice Profit and Loss Statement

of reimbursement. ACO distributions can replace professional fee revenue easily with no change in model structure. The key is then managing expenses based on the various forms of revenue available for generation. Thus, the model is very adaptable to moving toward value-based reimbursement.

The key challenge with this model is that it is the hardest to implement in a hospital-employed environment for a variety of factors, one of which is the higher expense structure in hospital-employed settings due to wage scales, occupancy costs, and other overhead items being higher. Further, the payer mix can change wherein professional fee revenue is less. These and other factors can result in the private practice style model not resulting in market compensation and thereby is perceived as untenable in a hospital-employed environment.

All of the information above is to highlight the fact that (1) the market has changed dramatically, (2) compensation model structures in hospital employment arrangements do not mirror that in private practice, and (3) as a result of points one and two, it requires real work to adapt compensation models to be relevant in the value-based realm, as is further described below.

Impact on wRVU Models

There is an overwhelming sense in the market that as value-based reimbursement ramps up, wRVU-based models will go by the wayside. While this may be true a long time into the future, wRVUs will have a place for many years to come in hospital-employed compensation models. This matter is especially the case for specialty care, where other than certain episodic initiatives, such as the Comprehensive Care for Joint Replacement or certain bundled payment pilots, fee-for-service reimbursement is still predominant. If wRVUs are still the primary means of reimbursement to align incentives, the compensation structure should be no different. Thus, until the market moves to a largely fully capitated model, wherein the capitation payments also include specialty care services, wRVU-based production will likely continue to play a role in the compensation strategy.

While primary care is somewhat different, wRVUs still play a role. With respect to primary care, wRVUs are being balanced out by a focus on patient panels. Patient panels are typically defined as unique patients seen by a physician in the last 18 months. A standard panel for a primary care physician averages around 1,800. Panel-based models are synonymous with capitation, wherein the revenue generated is not necessarily based on how much you do, but how many patients you manage. While there are pockets of capitation throughout the market, it is not yet a predominant reimbursement mechanism. Thus, fully moving a primary care model to panel size would be a bit premature.

With this in mind, once again, the incentive structure reverts back to wRVUs, as this is still driving reimbursement. That does not mean that panel cannot play a role in wRVU-based compensation models. In fact, it should begin to play a predominant role to (1) recognize the non-wRVU generating activities that are very much of a primary care physician's practice today, and (2) to ready practices for reimbursement models that are different than fee-for-service. Thus, often, wRVU production represents the majority of incentive, with panel becoming an ever-growing component. The trick will be to continue to balance these two components as the reimbursement model morphs over time.

Even if we wake up and find ourselves in a fully capitated market, that dynamic does not mean that wRVUs will go away. While they may not be the primary driver of incentive in a compensation model, it would still be reasonable to use them to measure what a physician is doing for the population of patients he or she is managing. Thus, wRVUs, while their use is evolving, will continue to play a role for the foreseeable future.

The Merit-Based Incentive Payment System (MIPS) that was put into effect as part of MACRA will undoubtedly have an impact on

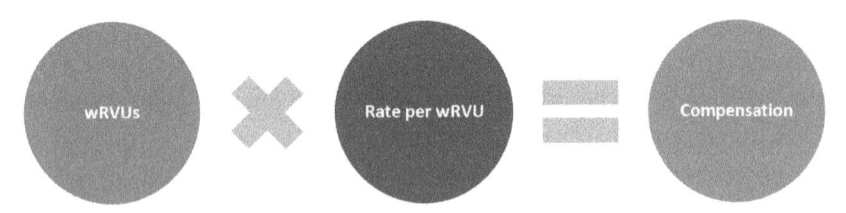

FIGURE 1.4.3 wRVU-Based Structure

wRVU-based compensation strategies in the future. Using Figure 1.4.3 as an example, pre-MIPS, the following was the typical wRVU-based structure.

The formula was rather simple. wRVUs were multiplied by a market-based compensation per wRVU ratio to derive compensation. Some models were more complex than this, but in its simplest form, this was the calculation. Thus, the only factor influencing compensation was how much a physician did, measured in wRVUs. With MIPS, this is no longer the case. While MIPS still focuses on how much a physician does, reimbursement is ultimately impacted by how well the work is performed. Thus, there are additional hurdles to jump through that affect ultimate reimbursement. In the context of a wRVU-based compensation model, the impact of MIPS can be illustrated in the following manner (see Figure 1.4.4, Rate per wRVU.)

The equation is very similar, but instead of the rate per wRVU being a constant, it is influenced by how well a physician performs in certain key non-productive areas. Thus, MIPS is a game changer with respect to reimbursement and should have the same effect on compensation arrangements. The effect of MIPS and other value-based arrangements are causing health systems to redesign their compensation arrangements in a variety of ways, which largely focuses on rebalancing the focus on production and performance. The appropriate balance is largely predicated on local reimbursement dynamics, with more aggressive markets

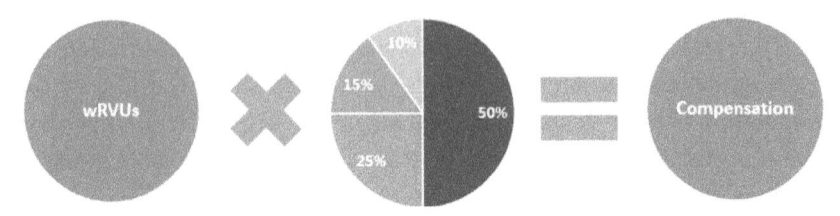

FIGURE 1.4.4 Rate per wRVU

pushing health systems to put more in the value/performance bucket, with the opposite not moving as quickly in this direction.

Overall, the balance of production and performance in the primary care realm tends to be a 70/30 to 85/15 split, with the former being the production focus and the latter being the performance/value focus. With specialty care, the split is more in the range of 85/15 to 95/5, with less of a focus on the value-based piece. This calculation is driven primarily by the market and less activity in the performance/value space for these specialties.

Influx of Panel-Based Incentives

Panel size has been mentioned numerous times throughout this chapter and rightfully so. It continues to play a larger role in the primary care compensation realm. If the market continues to move more toward capitation, panel will gain even more prominence.

The rationale for focusing on panel size is that it is indicative of the population of patients a primary care physician is responsible for managing on a day-to-day basis. Many payers are focused on how well the primary care physician cares for this population of patients and their overall health. Further, regardless of whether the physician is seeing these patients regularly in the office, he is responsible for taking care of their needs in terms of prescription refills, referrals to specialists, etc.

The goal of including panel size in compensation models is multi-faceted, as outlined below:

- **Encourage Access.** Incentives tied to panel size encourage physicians to maintain open panels, which helps to ensure that patients can have access to primary care physicians in their market and forces physicians to look at alternative means to expand access. This expansion is often through the use of advanced practice providers (APP) who can supplement what the physician is doing. In most panel incentives, the APP panels accrue to the physician to recognize his or her management of said panel. Alternatively, expansion can be through adding evening or weekend hours to make it more convenient for patients to come to see the physician.
- **Recognize Non-wRVU Producing Work.** Most primary care physicians would agree that the amount of non-patient facing work has grown tremendously over the last several years. This largely involves dealing with paperwork and other related matters

all tied to patient care but not separately reimbursement. By nature, the amount of this work grows as the panel size grows. Thus, including panel size in the compensation arrangement helps to recognize this added work, especially if it is in addition to a wRVU-based incentive.

- **Introduce Capitated Arrangements.** As mentioned, panel size is synonymous with capitation. Thus, include panel size in compensation arrangements when introducing the concept to physicians so if/when capitation grows, it will not be a shock. Further, much work goes into tracking panel size. Thus, simply by having it as a component of compensation forces the health system and physicians to pay attention to it, figure out how to best track and monitor it, etc.

Panel size can be introduced into compensation arrangements in a variety of manners. Some have a large impact on compensation and others have a smaller impact. Below, we highlight some options where panel size plays a role.

- **Derivation of Base Pay.** Some models let panel size drive the majority of compensation. For example, total compensation pay could be derived based on a per-member-per-month (PMPM) payment amount. For instance, total compensation could be derived using a PMPM amount of $10.50. Thus, an 1,800-panel size would equate to total compensation of $226,800. Of this amount, potentially $9.00 (approximately 85%) could be guaranteed, with the remaining $1.50 at risk based on performance metrics. Panel size would be reassessed quarterly with base pay reset for the following quarter. Such a model likely only makes sense if the reimbursement environment is largely capitated.
- **Small Add-On Component.** In other models, the panel size incentive is a small add-on component of compensation, representing 5% to 10% of total cash compensation. In these models, the economics of the panel size component is either established as an entirely separate component of pay or allocated as part of the overall value of pay. With respect to the former, it is simply a reduced calculation of that explained above. As an example, the panel component could be $1.50 PMPM, with this simply being an additional component of pay. As an example of the latter, consider

	wRVUs	Panel Size	Panel Incentive
Physician A	5,000	2,000	$8,000
Physician B	5,000	3,000	$12,000
	10,000	5,000	$20,000
Median Rate	$40.00		
Panel %	5%		
Panel Rate	$2.00		
Panel Pool	$20,000		

FIGURE 1.4.5 Panel-Based Compensation Arrangements

Figure 1.4.5. In this illustration, the targeted total compensation per wRVU is $40.00, with the panel component being worth $2.00 per wRVU. Thus, if two physicians generate 10,000 wRVUs, the panel pool is worth $20,000. This pool is then allocated out based on the physicians' respective panels. For example, Physician A has a panel of 2,000 and therefore gets 40% of the panel component, which equates to $4.00 per member (33 cents PMPM).

- **Allocation of Performance Incentive Opportunity.** Another way panel is introduced into a compensation model is in allocating the performance incentive opportunity. This example follows closely to that above, but instead of it simply being a direct payout to the physician, this sets the performance opportunity that the physician can earn, with the actual payout based on the physician's performance in that area. Using the above illustration as an example, Physician B's opportunity would have been $12,000. If he had scored a 75% on his performance scorecard, he would have been paid out $9,000.

While panel is being implemented in a variety of manners, the above highlights the fact that it is a growing focus in primary care compensation. This will continue to be the case as the reimbursement environment changes and payers continue to focus on primary care physicians improving the health of a population of patients.

The trickiest piece of including panel into a compensation arrangement is when the reimbursement market is a mix of capitation and fee-for-service. The approach to compensation under these two extremes is drastically different and requires different thought about compensation structures. Thus, having toes in both environments will be challenging at best, as patient care should not be different for one population vs. the other. In these environments, a bifurcated compensation approach may be necessary, with part of the model being wRVU-based and the rest being panel-based.

Treatment of External Incentives

A new phenomenon that exists with second generation compensation models is the fact that revenue sources have expanded to include more than just fee-for-service revenue. Now, there are other revenue streams from participation in ACO/CIN activities, shared savings models, governmental and commercial pay for performance programs, and others. A vital question about these new streams of revenue is what to do with them. In many cases, these programs start out small and then grow, meaning, in one year, there may be $500 to $1,000 attributed to a physician for his or her activity in a respective program.

In these instances, health systems have decided to treat these revenue streams as additional compensation and pass them through to the respective physician. While this is not always a problem, in the current environment, two factors have made this approach problematic.

The first challenge is that many compensation models were not designed to accommodate these additional incentives, which gets back to the "top-down" vs. "bottom-up" approach to compensation design discussed earlier. If the compensation model was not designed to have these funds passed through from a fair market value perspective, it could create potential compliance concerns. It is important to keep in mind that all of the market surveys used for compensation design and benchmarking, such as the Medical Group Management Association, American Medical Group Association, and Sullivan, Cotter and Associates, define their compensation benchmarks as total cash compensation (TCC)—that is, all forms of compensation that show up on a physician's IRS Form W-2 or K-1. Thus, if a physician is paid quality incentives, they would already be included in the metrics used to define TCC, meaning if the current compensation model is providing market-based compensation, these additional incentives should not necessarily be paid *on top of* the market-based compensation package.

The second challenge is the differentiation between revenue and compensation. As noted above, in many instances, these new forms of **revenue** are viewed as pass-throughs of additional **compensation.** There is a big different here. If value-based reimbursement is replacing fee-for-service reimbursement, then it is problematic to view these types of external incentives as compensation and not revenue. It sets the precedent that 100% of new forms of **revenue** will be passed through as additional **compensation.** Stepping back and considering this statement highlights the problematic nature of the situation. These funds should be viewed as new forms of revenue that then fund both overhead and the current compensation structure. They should not be passed through on-top-off. It is incumbent on the health system, from a compensation design standpoint, to ensure that the incentives in the compensation model are aligned with the incentives that drive value-based reimbursement—similar to what all health systems do with fee-for-service reimbursement in the sense that they use wRVUs or some other form of productivity as the primary incentive driver.

Typically, these incentive programs start out with $500 to $1,000 per physician, but they can quickly grow to something much more substantial. Further, often payers pay these funds as a true incentive at the onset of a program, but then quickly reduce fee-for-service reimbursement wherein to stay whole from a historical perspective, these value-based incentives must be captured. The Centers for Medicare and Medicaid Services (CMS) is notorious for structures like this. This phenomenon exacerbates the issues outlined above. Further, if a health system sets the precedent that these incentives are going to be passed through in the beginning and physicians get comfortable with the notion of such, changing course later on becomes even more difficult. Thus, it is important to treat these types of incentives right from the onset.

Balance of Incentives and Metrics

Second generation compensation models, by nature, are designed mainly with the premise of focusing on incentives outside of pure production. Thus, much focus is on quality, patient satisfaction, citizenship, cost control, etc. One reason health systems gravitate to production-based models is that they are easy to administer; the data points come from a single system and can be pulled together quite quickly. When metrics outside of production come into the equation, substantial work is required to gather the data for all of the other focus areas and turn them into something meaningful.

As was discussed in earlier chapters, this was an issue, but not a huge problem in first generation compensation models largely because (1) the incentive component was small ($5,000 to $15,000), and (2) the focus of the incentive was on less meaningful metrics. This issue is changing in second generation compensation models wherein (1) the value of the incentive is growing exponentially larger, and (2) the *desire* is to focus on more meaningful metrics.

As was mentioned earlier, for primary care, it is not uncommon to see health systems want to tie up to 25% of compensation to value-based metrics. With median primary care compensation being around $230,000, this means close to $60,000 can be tied to these metrics. The key question is what these funds should be tied to in order to justify the assigned value. This issue is a significant struggle, as physicians see these incentives as being riskier than production incentives and therefore want them tied to something meaningful, but something they can understand, they can track with accurate data, and they can influence directly. They feel that production incentives are largely in their control, meaning they either have the tools necessary to achieve the productivity incentives or they do not. This is not the case with value-based incentives and it mostly stems from a lack of data. While health systems spent millions of dollars implementing new medical records programs, this alone has not resulted in a wealth of data that can be used for value-based incentive metrics. The data may be in the programs, but the know-how to extract the data in a meaningful manner may not exist. Thus, health systems often are left with less-than-desirable metrics that they can accurately track or insufficient meaningful metrics that they want to track.

With this in mind, it is important for health systems to "grow into" these incentives. Moving from $5,000 of value tied to value-based metrics to $60,000 tied to value-based metrics overnight may be a lofty goal if the infrastructure is not there to support the move. While the $60,000 or more may be the ultimate aim, it is important to pace the implementation of these incentives based on the data available; otherwise, buy-in will be difficult. Further, it is important that health systems not limit themselves only to the incentive they can track or currently are tracking. Rather, they should define what they want to incentivize and determine what is needed to obtain those data. This matter will be more challenging and perhaps delay implementation of these incentives but should pay off in the end as the metrics will drive more change.

Finally, when considering value-based incentives, particularly as the amounts increase, it is important to balance the value of the incentives with the number of incentive metrics. Using an extreme example, it is not reasonable to tie $60,000 of value to a single patient satisfaction metric. At the same time, it is not reasonable to tie $8,000 to 15 different weight metrics. We recommend developing a scorecard that focuses on three or four key quality and patient satisfaction metrics for each specialty, one or two citizenship/access-related metrics, and then another one or two metrics important to group performance. The scorecard should be developed collaboratively among the physicians and the health system, and revisited annually to ensure that the metrics are still value-added to the health system.

CONCLUSION

Change is an operative word in healthcare today, and it is no less important when considering the activity in physician compensation arrangements. There is a dire need to ensure that incentives are aligned between a health systems' mission/vision/values, its reimbursement structure, and its physician compensation plan. With the reimbursement environment being ever evolving, this wreaks havoc in the stability of physician compensation arrangements, which must be adapted constantly to the rapidly changing market. While stability is desired, it may take a number of years for the current changes to flesh themselves out, which means that there is still more work to be done in adapting compensation models to meet the needs of the future reimbursement environment.

SECTION 1

CHAPTER 5

Negotiating Second Generation Contracts

INTRODUCTION

The contracts that were completed and executed three to five years ago are approaching their renewal dates. Most of those first generation contracts were between health systems/hospitals and physician groups under the auspices of productivity-based models. While those contracts did move the dial toward the physicians being at risk or having less guaranteed pay, they mainly focused on individual and/or group productivity. Further, the measurement of that productivity was almost always in work relative value units (wRVUs).

Now, several years later, as these original contracts are up for renewal, the negotiation process takes on a whole new look. Though productivity is still the focal point of these second generation contracts, there are other matters to consider based on the lessons learned from the first generation transactions.

The negotiation process is entirely relevant to these changes—some of which are obvious, while other issues are subtler. Those who are negotiating these renewal agreements, whatever their perspective, must be well versed on the positives and negatives of the original contracts, as well as the current and impending industry changes.

In this chapter, we will consider the essential tenets of the negotiation process relative to the second generation alignment contracts. First, we will discuss the critical issues in the process, followed by a review of the major components. Lastly, we will cover the keys to a successful second generation transaction.

Lessons Learned and Key Negotiation Considerations

As noted, the events that have occurred in recent years in the healthcare marketplace/industry have an enormous effect on second generation contracts. They require a thorough understanding of the experiences both in where the industry has moved since the negotiation and the consummation of the original transaction, and the direction that we anticipate we are heading before the expiration of the first generation deals. As a result, there are several significant points to address before entering the second generation negotiations.

- **Original contract positives and negatives.** A variety of first generation deals exist today. Some place most of their emphasis on workflow and the assignment of duties as opposed to requiring any level of productivity. Those contracts entail virtually all of the compensation to the providers as base pay; thus, the compensation is guaranteed. However, more of the existing contracts place emphasis on productivity as measured in wRVUs. The wRVUs are converted into compensation, usually based on a specific amount per wRVU and other key areas, mostly tied to financial performance. For example, many RVU values relate to costs based on the conversion factor of the previously private practicing physicians' actual wRVU take-home pay (that total amount relates to the overhead of the practice).

  Still, others emphasize a combination of productivity- and non-productivity-based incentives. However, in the final analysis, nearly all of the first generation contracts consider and place the providers at risk for their productivity and the resulting compensation.

  Realistically, these models could be interpreted as both pluses and minuses. Productivity is not a negative element of compensation when applied within proper legal and ethical parameters. However, as we move to a more value-based reimbursement system, the viability of productivity-based first generation contracts becomes less sustainable. What once was a positive facet of contracting might now be construed as a negative aspect.

  Other pluses and minuses of each first generation contract should be reviewed. It is the responsibility of both parties (i.e., the employer and the employee), and possibly an outside consul-

tant/advisor, to analyze and evaluate the good (and not-so-good) aspects of the first generation contracts to implement improvements in the second generation negotiations.
- **Changes in the reimbursement paradigm.** Clearly, the changes that have occurred and are expected in the future have a major effect on the second generation negotiation contract terms and conditions. As we move from volume to value reimbursement, the incentives must change as well as the entire financial/economic structure of the agreements. The contract negotiations must consider the impending changes, no matter the perspective (i.e., employer or employee). For example, as the bundled payments of reimbursement start to take shape, the metrics used to allocate monies from within the bundle to various providers are relevant to the contract going forward.
- **Structural changes.** Models of alignment vary, as they have since the initiation of the first generation contracts. Whether they are employment or even what we often call "employment lite" (i.e., professional services agreement [PSA] contracts), their structure going forward is relevant. We often are asked whether the financial terms should vary from a PSA to an employment model, and especially how they would be affected from the standpoint of a fair market value (FMV) or what is commercially reasonable (CR). In general, it should not matter whether the structure is a PSA or employment, the financial terms apply from a compliance standpoint with no difference in equivocating FMV and CR rates.

  However, structural changes are happening within the second generation models. For example, employment was often the original model, and it continues in the second generation, but many health systems recognize the value in allowing larger groups to remain autonomous and independent, especially in the day-to-day management. A model in use in the second generation contracts is the *group practice subsidiary* (GPS) model. While a legal subsidiary may or may not be created, the group is allowed to be structured and function as if it were a separate subsidiary with substantial day-to-day independence and autonomy. Technically, all of the providers, staff, etc., are still employed, but this structure is defined better within second generation models, as the negotiation process reflects.

(Note: Though the purpose of this chapter is not to sort out the various structures in second generation models [as discussed elsewhere], we should consider revisions to the structure in the context of the overall negotiations.)

- **Changes in terms and conditions.** The terms and conditions, often referred to as the mechanical or technical areas of the contract, may relate to various details about the term, renewal options, termination rights, restrictive covenants, exclusivity, indemnification, and myriad definitions and conditions to consider in the second generation contract. Though these issues were a part of the initial contract, the basic requirements must be revamped. They must reflect the structural, reimbursement, and compensation changes, as well as address the necessary adjustments in the relationships to meet the needs of the marketplace and to fit the current and forthcoming reimbursement parameters. Although the economic terms and revisions, plus some governance and leadership changes, are of the highest interest, contract renegotiations should consider the basic terms also.
- **Leadership and governance.** New contracts should expect to reflect changes in leadership and governance rights and obligations. The GPS model, noted above, is an example of how many groups are gaining more autonomy in day-to-day management and oversight. Likewise, PSA models typically entail a management committee comprising both health system and practice representatives (usually on an equal footing), with that committee as the governance and leadership body that oversees the PSA on a month-to-month basis. These types of arrangements should be investigated in the second generation negotiations to ensure all areas are covered, particularly with the changes under contemplation for the second generation contracts (i.e., structure, reimbursement, compensation incentives, terms and conditions, etc.).
- **Corporate considerations.** Another consideration whenever a health system and a practice are fully aligning through employment or PSA is the overall corporate oversight and management involvement within the health system. This factor also reflects on the cost allocations from the corporate management component of the health system down to the practice level. Analysis of the matters should be from an economic standpoint, and from gov-

ernance and leadership as well. The second generation contract negotiations must take into account any changes in the corporate structure since the initial contract negotiations and address them, as appropriate.

There are many elements to consider and to get right in the second generation contracts and the negotiation process in both economic and non-economic terms, regardless of the perspective. The review calls for a systematic and organized process that examines all the key points. One method is to develop a simple matrix to document the issues, i.e., an *issues tracker*. This tool will provide an organized effort from the perspectives of both sides to address all the issues; it also helps to identify those concerns that are most pressing and challenging. See Appendix A as an example of an issues tracker that we have used in actual work projects.

The Negotiation Process

The actual negotiation process for second generation contracts is similar to any other contract. However, the focus is on the key areas of consideration discussed in the previous section of this chapter. Following are descriptions of the specific tools to help facilitate the negotiation process.

- **Financial analysis.** Every negotiation process should encompass a thorough financial analysis, which should be completed (often by an independent party/consultant) on behalf of either or both sides of the negotiation. Preferably, each party should provide its own outside assistance to formulate its financial analysis. In some cases, hospitals will be able to accomplish this analysis with their in-house financial department, obtaining outside consultative assistance only as needed. Such a report will assimilate the main components of the economic terms going forward, and will serve as a basis for determining the parameters of FMV and CR rates. Further, it can also help the health system understand its return-on-investment parameters and realize the most economic forms of payment. This financial analysis should be developed in some detail, comparing historical performance during the first generation contract life, in terms of productivity of the providers (dollars and wRVUs), cost/overhead, and ultimately, the compensation derived. The health system must be careful not to tie any value of the downstream revenue to the physicians' compensation in the second generation contracts. This factor should not be a part of the financial analysis.

- **Issues tracker.** The issues tracker discussed in the previous section is valuable for the overall negotiation process. An example of an issues tracker is provided in Appendix A. Note that the issues are tracked with a "light/medium/dark gray" signification. The darkest gray designates the issues for which there is little agreement; the medium gray is for those that have the most agreement but some resolution remains; and the lightest gray are those that have been reconciled and agreement is reached.

  The issues tracker is an organization tool and, as the negotiations move along, it will eliminate all those areas that have been resolved and allow the parties to focus on those issues that remain.

- **Letter of intent.** The letter of intent (LOI) is an important document in that it encapsulates all the key terms and conditions—both economic and non-economic—relative to the second generation transaction. It should be updated as issues are resolved and may be used in a tracked form to identify the changes and to maintain a document that will ultimately be used to draft the definitive agreements. (See Appendix B for an example LOI.)

- **Definitive agreements.** Once the issues are resolved and the LOI agreed upon (if not fully executed), the final agreements will be drafted. Depending on the structure of the second generation alignment, the definitive agreements may entail nothing more than an employment contract or a PSA contract, possibly to include an asset purchase agreement. In more complicated cases where management services are being provided by the practice, there may be a practice support services agreement (PSSA). Also, at times there may be a management services agreement (MSA) that outlines the standard terms and conditions. We have provided examples of both a PSSA (Appendix C) and an MSA (Appendix D).

The negotiation process should involve a variety of tools, including documents that support the negotiations as a "work in process," working toward the final definitive agreements. Using these tools and maintaining organization are helpful for navigating the second generation negotiation process.

Keys to a Successful Second Generation Transaction

Other overarching points of consideration that lead to a successful negotiation of the second generation agreement are as follows:

- **Understand the process and the overall flow of negotiations.** The negotiation process is somewhat both an art and science in that both parties should be willing to do what it takes to complete the transaction. Often, it takes time and a spirit of "give and take" to work through some of the most difficult issues. Therefore, using the issues tracker presented earlier in this chapter is important, as it helps to improve the efficiency of the process and to zero in on the crucial areas of difference. Another means to help the parties strike a deal is to have a healthy respect for the ebb and flow of the negotiation process, with neither side overreacting or getting too caught up in the other side's positions.

   Also, it is important to engage outside advisors, including healthcare consultants and attorneys. These are professionals who will separate the personal (and even emotional) feelings that are inevitably at play among the two parties of the transaction. A primary objective of developing these second generation contracts is making sure to address all areas, even the more difficult ones, while not generating negative feelings in the working relationship, post-transaction.

- **Respect the changes in the industry.** Many people falsely assume that the second generation deal should be easy and without major hiccups, based on the first generation contract. This assumption is unrealistic due to the striking changes in the healthcare industry that must be factored into the second generation contract.

   Moreover, these adjustments are happening slowly, which is a factor that becomes even more challenging as the second generation contract negotiations continue with a near-term effective date. In contrast, many of the modifications in the industry (such as volume-to-value reimbursement) are far from fully defined, much less established, which minimizes the effect on the new contracts.

- **Delineate the key needs and expectations of both parties.** Sometimes the unstated or less-than-fully-explained points lead to the greatest areas of confusion, distrust, and polarity. Thus, it is important that both sides fully articulate the crucial areas relative to their needs and expectations, perhaps even to the point of drawing some lines in the sand. A lack of clarity tends to breed distrust and uncertainty, which has the potential for undermining the transaction. It is essential to have a precise definition of each side's position, along with a spirit of compromise.
- **Create a negotiation subgroup.** Depending on the size of the organizations, it is much better to "boil down" the negotiation process to a smaller group of representatives from both sides. These representatives should include outside advisors/legal counsel and be limited to decision makers or their designees within each organization. Those who are designated to represent the decision makers should have close access to those who can make decisions rapidly.

  Using a subgroup process is efficient, and it allows for better timing and an enhanced approach toward completion. Those who are within the direct negotiation subgroup should communicate to others in their organization, keeping them informed of the negotiation process and obtaining direction and supervision, as applicable.
- **Avoid misunderstandings at all times.** The likelihood of misunderstanding and delay (and possible negation) of the negotiation process is high without the documentation of those things that have been agreed upon (as by using an issues tracker tool and/or recording in a LOI). The negotiation is a spirited process that often results in amplified emotions. And, because so much of the discussion involves economic terms over many years in the future, it rightfully takes on added significance. In short, proper documentation eliminates misunderstandings. Often, people hear things differently as opposed to reading what is in writing, and avoiding disputes is essential to successful second generation contract negotiations. This same caution goes for mixed messages that include incomplete responses or perhaps, worse, incomplete answers to all points. (For example, if a party is not ready to respond to a particularly point in the negotiations, they should

acknowledge that they are not ready rather than pass over and ignore the matter.)
- **Allow for changes in the future, post-transaction.** No one knows how the future in healthcare and reimbursement structures will unfold and what issues will be pertinent to the second generation alignment contracts. It is wise, therefore, and essential, perhaps, to allow for some areas of change and/or adjustment as the industry sorts through various issues and clarifies what will transpire. This flexibility particularly pertains to the reimbursement structures and how fast we will move away from fee-for-volume versus fee-for-value. Then, how soon will we need to adjust the compensation incentive structures of employed or contracted providers with health systems and/or other entities? Often, the agreement stipulates that if a certain percentage of the total reimbursement changes, further discussion and the possible reopening of negotiations for revisions to the contract is all that is necessary to occur. Moreover, adding a requirement for some form or timeframe for transitioning is entirely appropriate, rather than forcing an overnight change.

CONCLUSION

The keys to successful negotiation of the second generation contract ultimately may be summarized in a simple statement that the process should be collaborative, communicative, and transparent. With these characteristics in play, along with a give-and-take spirit by both parties, the likelihood of a successful second generation contract increases.

ABC PRACTICE ("ABC" AND/OR THE "PRACTICE") AND DEF HEALTH ("DEF" AND/OR "SYSTEM") (COLLECTIVELY, THE "PARTIES"): LETTERS OF INTENT COMPARATIVE REVIEW

Upon review of DEF's latest response/term sheet received on DATE, we believe their current offer is a continued improvement from the previous transactional structure. ABC's Board approved the Term Sheet with minor revisions. Nevertheless, we believe that further clarification is necessary before an enactment of agreement (at least, before the execution of any formal agreements). Much of the need for additional clarity is the fact that the latest DEF Term Sheet omits various previously presented and/or agreed upon terms. We note these areas and the status of all transactional components within the table below.

Also, we note that ABC responded to DEF's DATE Term Sheet by "red-lining" unacceptable/additional terms. Therefore, if a term was left unchanged by ABC, we have assumed that ABC has accepted the appropriate DEF response; hence, we have removed that term from the tracker and have considered it resolved. Further, we note that DEF's DATE Term Sheet, as well as their DATE Term Sheet, have omitted several terms that were a part of DEF's previous LOI, many of which, in Coker's opinion, are important to the overall agreement and merit further discussion and/or resolution. Thus, we do not consider the DATE Term Sheet representative of the entire transaction, but rather that DEF's DATE Term Sheet indicates the high-level points of a final agreement.

We have updated the original tracker to reflect only those terms that require further discussion (either internally and/or with DEF).

Ultimately, we defer to ABC as to final determination for these remaining points. We merely note/highlight them to assure their consideration.

Terms reflected in DATE DEF Term Sheet considered Resolved (not reflected in tracker):	Terms not reflected in the DATE DEF Term Sheet but agreed upon previously (in the previous LOI) (not reflected in tracker)
• Providers • Term of Agreement • Extension of Agreement • Termination • Practice Liabilities • Income Distribution Plan • Services at non-DEF's Facilities • Management Functions • Billing and Collections • Practice Physician Services • Purchase of Practice Assets • Excluded Assets • Professional and Technical Fees • Payment to the Practice • PSA Global Rates • Real Estate Leases • DEF Responsibilities • Permitted Outside Activities • Independence	• Marketing and Branding • Strategy for Tertiary Market Penetration • Collaboration on Reimbursement Initiatives • New Technology • Existing Technology • Duties, Space, Equipment and Personnel • FMV and CR Reports • Dispute Resolution • Other Terms and Conditions

Note: We request ABC management to review the above summary and assure proper disposition of all terms/conditions.

Terms *not* addressed in the DATE DEF Term Sheet but further discussion/resolution required (highlighted in light gray)	Terms addressed in the DATE DEF Term Sheet but further discussion/agreement required (highlighted in medium gray)	Terms addressed in the DATE DEF Term Sheet, but significant disagreement exists (highlighted in dark gray)
• Unwind • Minimum Income Guarantee • Exclusivity and Right of First Refusal • Indemnification • Exclusivity • Restrictions on Physicians Who Leave the Practice • Pass-through of Performance Dollars	• Ownership and Practice Overhead • Practice Overhead Reimbursement • Ancillary Equipment Lease • Ancillary Overhead Pass-through • Management Committee • Non-Compete Arrangement • Ownership and Practice Overhead • Practice Overhead Reimbursement	• Structure of Proposed Transaction in General

Note: We recommend Coker and ABC review the tracker collaboratively and ensure internal agreement on the major points of this transaction. Upon the achievement of a consensus, we will examine the definitive agreements delivered to ABC on behalf of DEF to ensure all appropriate and acceptable terms are reflected. We will continue to assist in the implementation, and other phases as ABC directs (see the separate summary of "Next Steps/Tasks to be Completed").

Appendix A 65

Term/Condition	ABC LOI	DEF Response	ABC/Coker Response/Counterproposal
1. Proposed Transaction in General	PSA with ABC remaining separate from GHI	PSA with ABC as a separate operational unit with ____ ("ABC Section"), with an independent shared operational responsibility and governance. Deleted Term: "The GHI Board of Directors would not have jurisdiction over the ABC Section. The ABC Section within GHI is established exclusively for payer contracting and credentialing and operational decision-making, and governance will be exclusively restricted to . . ." Added term: While the ABC Section would be an operational unit under the corporate structure of GHI, the manner in which the ABC Section would be operated and governed would be agreed upon by the parties and outlined in the PSA. In particular, the governance model would include the elements described in the "Independence," "Corporate Governance Committee," and "DEF Responsibilities" sections, and the joint operating committee would serve as the focal point for the relationship between the parties.	We believe this requires further discussion.
2. Unwind	Parties can mutually agree to unwind and return to pre-PSA status after three years of the PSA; ABC would have the first right of refusal to reacquire sold assets.	Parties can mutually agree to unwind and return to pre-PSA status following termination; ABC will have the right of refusal for sold assets and transferred leases.	This matter was not addressed in DEF's Term Sheet but should be included as a term, particularly in the definitive agreements, as it will allow both parties to terminate the agreement mutually at any time during the contract. The practical effect of the Term, Termination, and Restrictive Covenant sections would allow for a permissible unwind; however, this provision should still be stated explicitly in any final agreement.

Term/Condition	ABC LOI	DEF Response	ABC/Coker Response/Counterproposal
3. Ownership and Practice Overhead	Practice will retain ownership of Practice entity and assets; ABC will be responsible for managing overhead expenses and administrative infrastructure of the Practice, which could include the leasing o ancillary staff to DEF.	While the ABC Section would be an operational unit under the corporate structure of DEF, the manner in which the ABC Section would be operated and governed would be agreed upon by the parties and outlined in the PSA. In particular, the governance model would include the elements described in the "Collaborative Practice Operations" section below; the joint operating committee would serve as the focal point for the relationship between the parties. DEF would ultimately be responsible for the reasonable costs of all space, staff, equipment, marketing, and other overhead required for the operation of the ABC Section (including reimbursing ABC for staff and overhead provided by ABC and related entities). Estimated (budgeted) overhead expense reimbursement would be paid on a monthly basis, subject to quarterly and year-end reconciliation based on actual expenses. The parties would identify day-to-day operational and physician issues that would continue to be overseen by Practice Physicians. Practice Physician issues would include day-to-day clinical practice operations. Additionally, the Practice would remain responsible for: • Internal corporate governance; • Internal ABC finance, taxes, and budgeting; • Income distribution among Practice Physicians; and • Accounts payable (i.e., ABC expenses).	ABC has agreed with DEF's response. However, with respect to the costs associated with the Practice responsibilities, the operating budget should incorporate for such reimbursements by DEF, and the payment should be based upon the budgeted total except for variable expenses. Needs further clarity.

Appendix A   **67**

Term/Condition	ABC LOI	DEF Response	ABC/Coker Response/Counterproposal
4. Practice Overhead Reimbursement and Other Services	ABC will be reimbursed for fixed overhead costs per a budgeted amount per year and for variable overhead costs as a rate per wRVU.	**Overhead Reimbursement:** The Practice receives overhead reimbursement for staff and other overhead expenses that are set forth in a budget approved by the PSA Management Committee. Practice will manage such overhead expenses within the budget. The overhead reimbursement to Practice will be based on Practice's actual costs for such staff and other budgeted expenses. Added term: Estimated (budgeted) overhead expense reimbursement would be paid on a monthly basis, subject to quarterly and year-end reconciliation based on actual expenses. Other Services: In the event DEF requests that Practice provide services in new geographies, or that Practice relocate services or providers, or if the parties pursue new ventures through the PSA that do not involve wRVU generating services, the parties will negotiate the compensation for such services to be reflected in an amendment to the PSA.	This section requires further discussion as the overhead expense reimbursement should be based upon the budgeted total except for variable expenses. ABC has accepted DEF's Response to "Other Services."
5. Ancillary Equipment Lease and Overhead Pass-Through	Subject to the Practice's discretion, DEF would lease certain ancillary leases at a **TBD** fair market value rate with all OH costs reimbursed as pass-throughs.	Term removed by DEF to align with total asset purchase	This matter requires further discussion and is contingent on the Practice's decision to sell all assets. Ideally, all lease assignments would pass through in the overhead reimbursement category.
6. Pass-Through of Performance Dollars	ABC will retain 100% of CPCI dollars and other performance revenue as a pass-through.	Term removed with request for all such dollars to be retained by DEF under "Professional and Technical Fees" term.	This item was not mentioned in DEF's Term Sheet, but this matter should be addressed in the form of the adjusted wRVU rates previously discussed.*

Term/Condition	ABC LOI	DEF Response	ABC/Coker Response/Counterproposal
7. Minimum Income Guarantee	DEF to provide an income guarantee for first 3 years of PSA equal to 80% of the Providers' historical 3-year production average.	Term removed	This matter was not addressed in DEF's Term Sheet, and we believe it warrants further consideration and commitment from DEF to not decrease the Practice's compensation from historical levels.
8. Management Committee	Joint governing body of 3 ABC appointed representatives (not subject to DEF approval) and 3 DEF personnel (one administrator and two physicians). The Agreement will fall under the Hospital's purview and not be a part of GHI. The committee will be driven by a majority voting structure with DEF retaining certain reserved powers.	Parties would establish a joint operating committee to address issues of mutual interest regarding the ABC Section, including: • Marketing and advertising • Strategic Planning • Consultation regarding payer contracting • ABC Section budget • Medical management for the ABC Section • Capital and other expenditures • Physician recruitment • [Added term] New services for the ABC Section ABC may appoint an internal ABC medical director who shall coordinate efforts with DEF chief medical officer. DEF will not limit or control the ABC Physicians' independent clinical judgment, provided all services will be performed in accordance with applicable standards of care.	This item appears acceptable, as well; however, how the applicable standards of care will be determined should be discussed.

*Alternatively, the rate per wRVU may be the implicit intent of DEF to mitigate the lack of pass-through of performance funds. ABC should now clarify this position.

Appendix A **69**

Term/Condition	ABC LOI	DEF Response	ABC/Coker Response/Counterproposal
9. Non-Compete	The PSA will not entail a non-compete.	Non-compete for 2 years after termination or the date Physician ceases services under PSA within the circular areas centered on the Practice's then existing offices, each having a radius of fifteen (15) miles; Physician/Practice can return to private practice following termination. The restrictive covenants would not apply in the event of (a) termination by Practice due to DEF breach; (b) termination by DEF without cause, or (c) non-renewal by DEF. The parties recognize that the restrictive covenants must apply to individual Practice Physicians. DEF and ABC would explore how best to accomplish this matter, which may include an evaluation of existing ABC non-competes.	It appears that ABC has agreed with DEF's Response. We still believe a two-year term is excessive but understand that DEF is unlikely to flex on this timeframe. ABC should now sign off on this stipulation.
10. Exclusivity and First Right of Refusal (ROFR)	Practice will be preferred providers of DEF; system will not engage other family practitioners to join GHI who will compete with ABC's service lines; recruitment subject to community needs analysis (CNA) with Practice having ROFR on new physicians.	Removed preferred provider, CNA language, and ROFR language. Recruitment will be discussed through the Management Committee and mutually agreed upon; replacement physician language relatively consistent.	While the Term Sheet alludes to this term, the actual definitive agreement should include ROFR language that allows the Practice to have the first right of refusal to repurchase all sold assets and re-employ support staff following an unwind. These items would include all assets sold at the time of the date of closing and all new assets acquired by the Hospital during the Term of the Agreement.

Term/Condition	ABC LOI	DEF Response	ABC/Coker Response/Counterproposal
11. Restrictions on Physicians Who Leave the Practice	Departed Physicians would be subject to a 12-month exclusivity period with DEF and any such confidentiality agreements.	Departed Physicians would be subject to a 12-month exclusivity period with DEF, the non-compete restrictions and any such confidentiality agreements.	This matter was not addressed in DEF's DATE Term Sheet, although the Term Sheet does state that departing Practice Physicians would be subject to the non-compete provision. More clarity regarding this provision should be sought.
12. Indemnification	DEF agrees to indemnify the Practice.	Term removed.	This item was not addressed in DEF's Term Sheet. We believe this language should be reinserted in the LOI and reflected in the definitive agreement.
13. Exclusivity	N/A	From the date of this LOI until the earlier of DATE or the date DEF has notified Practice in writing that it is no longer interested in proceeding with the PSA, Practice shall negotiate exclusively with DEF and shall not engage in or cooperate with any person or entity with respect to any (i) merger, sale of assets, sale of or tender offer for equity interest of or similar transactions involving Practice, or (ii) direct or indirect employment of or independent contract with Practice's physicians, in each case other than with DEF.	This issue was not addressed in DEF's Term Sheet, and we believe it should be resolved to avoid ABC indirectly agreeing to a DATE exclusivity period. We recommend "closing the loop" on this matter with agreeing to an extended exclusivity period, if the parties demonstrate mutual agreement/resolution on a vast majority of the key terms (including the economics) by DATE. Thus, DATE will serve as a "checkpoint" for the parties to assess progress and the overall likelihood of completing the transaction in a mutually agreeable manner.

APPENDIX B

— CONFIDENTIAL —

SUMMARY OF KEY TERMS OF THE
PROPOSED PHYSICIAN EMPLOYMENT AGREEMENTS
BETWEEN THE PHYSICIANS ("PHYSICIANS") OF ABC PRACTICE, P.C., (THE "PRACTICE") AND
DEF PHYSICIAN GROUP, d.b.a. GHI MEDICAL GROUP ("GHI")

This summary ("Summary") memorializes the key terms of the Physicians' "second generation" employment agreements (hereafter, the "Agreement") with GHI and documents the mutually agreeable go-forward transaction structure. This document reflects both economic and non-economic provisions agreed upon by the Practice and GHI to-date. The Practice and GHI are collectively referred to as the "Parties" herein. This is not intended to be all inclusive, meaning that only primary points within the anticipated new employment agreements are noted. The definitive agreements will entail all applicable matters.

1. **Term of Agreement:** Initial term of five years

2. **Extension of Agreement:** Automatic extensions for consecutive one year terms ("Extension Term") upon the expiration of the Initial Term or applicable Extension Term unless either Party terminates the Agreement per the final agreed upon termination provisions.

3. **Termination:** Either Party may terminate the Agreement (without cause) after 36 months following the Effective Date by providing a 365-day written notification; standard with cause termination provisions apply.

4. **Unwind:** In the event of an unwind, the Practice will have the right of first refusal to acquire assets that support the Physicians at the then fair market value (as determined by a mutually agreed upon third party), and directly employ its support staff, as applicable.

5. **Support Staff:** All Practice support staff and administrators will remain employees of St. Francis Health System and receive compensation and benefits equal to or higher than historical rates. No breaks in service will result (from the current employment to the subsequent employment resulting from the physicians' new contracts).

6. **Ancillary Services and Equipment:** The Practice will retain ownership of all assets related to the ancillary services, which will remain on-site at a Practice location at all times. GHI will lease these assets at FMV throughout the Initial Term and any Extension Terms. All revenue generated therefrom will belong to GHI, but will continue to be billed under standard professional rates (not HOPD).

7. **Compensation – Base Salary:** Payable in equal bi-weekly installments across twenty-six (26) pay periods per year, in keeping with GHI's standard pay practices. If the wRVU production threshold yields a negative remainder for the aggregate of two (2) consecutive complete calendar quarters after the first year of employment, GHI will have the option to reduce Base Salary for the remainder of the Initial Term to a level equivalent of annualized wRVUs multiplied by the conversion rate. Thus, the Base Salary is not guaranteed, but predicated on the successful achievement of a minimum wRVU threshold.

8. **Compensation – Production:** GHI will remit payment to each Physician[1] based upon their individual wRVU productivity. Compensation will be calculated using a single-tier rate per wRVU value of $57.50. An overview of the overall compensation methodology can be seen below.

Rate/wRVU Components	Year 1	Year 2	Year 3	Year 4**	Year 5**
Total Rate/wRVU	$57.50	$58.65	$59.82	$61.02	$62.24
Production*	$55.78	$56.89	$58.03	$57.97	$59.13
Total Incentive	$1.73	$1.76	$1.79	$3.05	$3.11
Guaranteed Incentive	$1.73	$1.76	$1.79	$1.53	$1.56
At Risk	$0.00	$0.00	$0.00	$1.53	$1.56
Total Guaranteed Rate/wRVU	$57.50	$58.65	$59.82	$59.49	$60.68

*The production piece for years 1-3 is 97% of the total rate/wRVU, with no portion of the incentive being at risk. Starting in Year 4, the production portion of the rate/wRVU drops to 95% of the total, with the remaining 5% tied to the incentive piece, and 2.5% of the total rate/wRVU is considered at-risk.

**Assumes a maximum increase in the Production-only wRVU compensation rate of 2% year-over-year for Years 4 and 5

Dr. Doe is excluded from this methodology and will be compensated consistent with historical practice (i.e. via a fixed salary with the potential for an incentive bonus each year). The remainder of Physicians will share in a distribution each year of the $70,000 related to their assumption of duties on behalf of the non-1.0 FTE Physician workforce.

Beginning in year four, an annual adjustment factor will be applied to the targeted effective comp/wRVU to account for environmental changes and will be subject to an adjustment collar (both up and down) to limit significant year-over-year fluctuations in compensation. The collars limit the max year-over-year change (up and down) to 2.0 percent unless a material change in per unit reimbursement occurs. A material change in reimbursement will be defined as 15 percent or greater. Should a material change in reimbursement occur, the parties will have the option of renegotiating the contract.

Employment agreement terms will set forth the process to reconcile employment and physician compensation should a material change in reimbursement occur. Determinants of the annual adjustment factor will be physician compensation benchmark surveys and contracted payor rates.

A more detailed summary with examples will be included within the definitive agreements.

9. **Compensation – Performance Incentive:** For the first three years of the Agreement, the Physicians' will be guaranteed incentive dollars totaling 3% of their projected total compensation for the achievement of mutually agreeable performance measures, paid on a quarterly basis. The scope of the performance incentive will be increased to five percent in Years 4 and 5 with 2.5% of the 5% guaranteed.

10. **Compensation – Call Penalty:** Consistent with current practice, the reduction in compensation incurred by those Physicians who do not take call will be used to fund a pool of monies, which will then be distributed equally amongst the Physicians who do participate in call on a semi-annual basis.

11. **Compensation – Call Buy-back:** Physicians choosing to work either the morning after call or their afternoon off will be compensated $750.

12. **Compensation – Back-up call:** Physicians receive $300 per day while providing back-up call coverage and $500 per day when called to present while on back-up call.

13. **Benefits:** GHI will provide the Physicians with a comprehensive benefits package that is consistent with that offered to similarly situated physicians and equal to or higher than historical levels.

14. **Medical Directorship Stipend:** The existing medical directorship arrangements will remain with payment for same occurring independent of the professional services' compensation. The Parties acknowledge that St. Francis Health System's evaluation of administrative roles and medical directorships may ultimately impact the current medical directorship arrangements.

15. **Governance:** The governance structure will be consistent with that documented within the POC Charter and ultimately included within the definitive agreements.

16. **IT Infrastructure:** The Practice will integrate with GHI's IT platform by implementing EPIC as its new electronic health record and practice management systems. This is anticipated to occur in February, 2016.

17. **EPIC Protection:** During the transition period and commencing immediately after the effective date of implementation, GHI will provide each Physician with income protection for a period of forty (40) clinic days (i.e., GHI will make each Physician "whole" for any lost productivity that results from the transition during the 40-clinic day period). Further clarification as to the exact mechanics and economics of this will be included within the definitive agreements.

18. **Services at Non-St. Francis-Owned Facilities**: The Physicians will not be prohibited from continuing to provide services at Greenville Health System.

In addition to the points above, there are several outstanding issues that require resolution. These include:

19. **Research:** The parties are in agreement that the proceeds from research to the Physicians will be treated on a "bottom line" basis. However, the allocation of revenue and expenses for the research component needs to be vetted.

This Summary is intended to outline the proposed terms of an affiliation and to further the ongoing discussions between the Parties. This Summary is not, and is not intended to be, a binding agreement on the part of any Party, nor does it create any obligation or liability on the part of any Party. The Parties acknowledge that this letter does not contain all the material terms and conditions of a binding agreement with respect to the matters currently under discussion, and that no binding agreement will exist between them with respect to the matters discussed in this Summary until all parties have executed the written definitive agreement(s) with respect to the matters described therein.

Acknowledged and Agreed:

_____   _____
ABC PRACTICE, P.C.   DATE

_____   _____
GHI MEDICAL GROUP   DATE

APPENDIX C

PROFESSIONAL SERVICES AGREEMENT FOR SPECIALTY SERVICES

This **PROFESSIONAL SERVICES AGREEMENT** (this "**Agreement**") is entered into on _____, 2016, to be effective as of _____, 2016 (the "**Effective Date**"), by and among DEF Hospital, a STATE nonprofit corporation ("**DEF**"), GHI Clinical Services, a STATE nonprofit corporation affiliated with DEF ("**GHI**"), and ABC Specialty Practice, P.A., a STATE professional association ("**ABC**"). GHI and ABC are sometimes collectively referred to herein as the "**parties**" and individually as a "**party**."

RECITALS

WHEREAS, DEF owns acute care hospitals located at [_____] and [_____] (collectively the "**Hospitals**" and each a "**Hospital**"), in which it provides inpatient and outpatient SPECIALTY services to the community (collectively "**SPECIALTY Services**");

WHEREAS, ABC is a medical professional association that employs physicians with the qualifications, expertise and experience to provide professional services for DEF with regard to SPECIALTY Services;

WHEREAS, DEF, in furtherance of its charitable mission and with the intention of providing a community benefit, has formed GHI for the purpose of contracting with ABC to provide SPECIALTY Services to DEF patients in order to improve the availability of quality professional medical services to the community served by DEF and the Hospitals;

WHEREAS, GHI and ABC have determined that it is desirable to coordinate and integrate the provision of SPECIALTY Services in order to improve the quality, efficiency and reputation of these services; and

WHEREAS, ABC is willing to enter into this Agreement with GHI and DEF, together with a Practice Support Services Agreement ("**PSSA**"), Lease of Assets ("**Asset Lease**"), Lease for Second Floor of ABC Building ("**New Programs Lease**"), SPECIALTY Service Line Management Services Agreement ("**MSA**") (collectively, the "**Transaction Agreements**") and perform the SPECIALTY Services set forth herein on the terms and conditions herein stated.

AGREEMENT

NOW, THEREFORE, in consideration of the above recitals, which recitals are hereby incorporated in and made a part of this Agreement, the mutual covenants and agreements contained herein and for other good and valuable consideration, the receipt and sufficiency of which is acknowledged by the parties, the parties agree as follows:

ARTICLE 1
ABC'S RIGHTS AND RESPONSIBILITIES

Section 1.1. Engagement.

(a) GHI hereby engages ABC, and ABC hereby accepts such engagement, to provide the SPECIALTY Services in accordance with the terms and conditions of this Agreement. Notwithstanding the foregoing, the engagement does not include the services that are identified on Exhibit 1.1(a) (the "**Excluded Services**").

(b) In carrying out its duties hereunder, ABC shall be an independent contractor of DEF and GHI. ABC shall be subject to the standards and terms set forth in this Agreement. Neither this Agreement nor the exercise of any of the authority granted to ABC hereunder shall be deemed to create any partnership, joint venture, association or other relationship among ABC, GHI and DEF other than that of an independent contractor relationship.

(c) DEF and GHI do not and shall not engage in the practice of medicine. Each physician employee of ABC who provides professional services hereunder shall exercise his or her own independent professional judgment in the care and treatment of the patients and DEF, GHI, ABC shall not interfere with each such physician's exercise of professional medical judgment; provided, however, that the services to be provided hereunder by ABC shall be provided in a manner consistent with the professional standards governing such services and the provisions of this agreement.

Section 1.2. Responsibilities of ABC.

(a) Commencing on the Effective Date and continuing through the Term of this Agreement, ABC, through those physicians (collectively, the "**Physicians**") set forth on Exhibit 1.2(a) (which such exhibit shall be updated promptly by ABC upon written notice to GHI, including without limitation updates necessary to reflect newly-added physicians to ABC), shall provide SPECIALTY Services on behalf of GHI, subject only to the expressed limitations herein set forth. ABC shall carry out its duties and obligations in a professional and competent manner consistent with good business practices.

(b) ABC shall cause the Physicians, collectively, to provide services on a full-time basis, twenty-four hours a day, seven days a week, and three hundred sixty-five days per year, including specifically SPECIALTY coverage for patients presenting to the Emergency Department of DEF pursuant to such protocols and standards as shall be established from time to time.

(c) ABC shall cause each Physician to agree, in writing, to reassign such Physician's professional revenue to DEF and to execute a reassignment in the form of *Exhibit 1.2(c)* hereto. The parties acknowledge that pursuant to a separate Transaction Agreement, ABC shall bill and collect, on behalf of DEF and as DEF's agent, the income for SPECIALTY Services rendered by the Physicians to patients, regardless of where such services are provided. Except as specifically permitted hereby, neither ABC nor any of its Physicians shall submit claims or otherwise attempt to collect for such services. In the event that any Physician is not able to effectively assign any such amounts to DEF, ABC shall collect such amounts and shall pay over any such amounts daily to DEF.

(d) ABC acknowledges that DEF is a charitable corporation to be operated in a manner that furthers charitable purposes by promoting health for a broad cross-section of the community and in compliance with the standards articulated by the Internal Revenue Service for tax-exempt health care organizations. ABC shall perform its services in compliance with DEF's charity care policies and stated mission and purpose, to include providing quality health services to all patients needing such services without regard to race, creed, color, religion, national origin, disability, gender, sexual orientation, insurance coverage or ability to pay.

(e) The SPECIALTY Services provided by ABC to GHI shall meet the standards of the community for such services.

(f) ABC agrees to comply with and cause each of its Physicians and employees providing services hereunder to comply with DEF's reasonable administrative and utilization review/quality management, integrity, and compliance policies.

Section 1.3. Qualifications of ABC Physicians. Throughout the Term of this Agreement, ABC shall ensure that each Physician providing services hereunder shall:

(a) Execute a reassignment in the form of Exhibit 1.2(c);

(b) Maintain an unrestricted license to practice medicine in the State of STATE and dispense prescription medications;

(c) Be a member in good standing of the Hospital's Medical Staff and, if specified as necessary to perform services under this Agreement, be a member in good standing at one or more additional facilities as designated by DEF, with status in the active category with appropriate clinical privileges;

(d) Be board-certified or board-eligible in SPECIALTY;

(e) Maintain participating provider status with Medicare and Medicaid programs and not have been deemed excluded from participation in any federally funded health care program, including but not limited to Medicare and Medicaid;

(f) Maintain the insurance required by Section 5.3 of this Agreement;

(g) Maintain an unrestricted federal DEA registration and any applicable state permits; and

Section 1.4. Failure to Meet Qualifications. ABC shall notify DEF within three (3) business days if any Physician no longer meets any of the foregoing requirements of Section 1.3. If any Physician or other person providing services hereunder fails to fulfill or otherwise abide by the requirements set forth in this Agreement, such person shall be excluded by ABC from the performance of services pursuant to this Agreement until such time as he or she again fulfills such requirements and, where applicable, is reinstated in accordance with the provisions of the Medical Staff Bylaws. During the time a Physician is excluded by ABC, the aggregate compensation under the terms of this Agreement shall be reduced accordingly.

Section 1.5. ABC Assets and Control. Except as expressly set forth in this Agreement or another Transaction Agreement, ABC and its shareholders shall:

(a) Retain full ownership of ABC and all assets associated with ABC;

(b) Retain full responsibility with regard to managing ABC's overhead expenses, subject to the budget approval process set forth in the PSSA; and

(c) Retain responsibility for all administrative services of ABC, subject to the terms of the PSSA.

ARTICLE II
DEF'S RIGHTS AND RESPONSIBILITIES

Section 2.1. Billing and Collection. DEF shall have the sole authority and responsibility for billing, collecting and retaining the income for the facility services rendered to DEF's patients; <u>provided, however</u> that the parties acknowledge that pursuant to the PSSA, ABC shall bill and collect, on behalf of DEF and as DEF's agent, the income for SPECIALTY Services rendered by the Physicians to patients, regardless of where such services are provided. DEF will negotiate all payer contracts and have responsibility for establishing fee schedules and reimbursement and payer strategies. ABC shall have the opportunity to provide input as to fee schedules and payer contracts, but the ultimate responsibility for such will be DEF's.

Section 2.2. Communications and Intellectual Property.

(a) The parties, through the Executive Committee (hereinafter defined) will agree upon a strategy for external communications regarding the SPECIALTY Services and this Agreement, including press releases, oral or written interviews or statements to the press and third-party payers.

(b) The parties, through the Executive Committee, will agree upon appropriate names, trademarks and other intellectual property to be identified with and utilized in the marketing of the SPECIALTY Services. Given ABC's long-standing presence in the CITY community and its strong brand recognition, the ABC name will be utilized to the greatest extent possible. Such intellectual property, excluding the ABC name, will be owned by DEF, and if registered, will be registered in the name of DEF. However, ABC will be permitted to use all such intellectual property for appropriate purposes during the Term of this Agreement, and for the purpose of notifying and informing patients only, for a period of six (6) months after termination of this Agreement. In the event of termination of this Agreement, no party will make any further use of the trademarks, trade names or other intellectual property utilized during the Term of this Agreement. All marketing and branding of pertinent services by DEF will be completed equally for ABC and other aligned practices. Notwithstanding anything to the contrary in this Agreement, DEF and ABC each retain all rights to their names as registered with the STATE Secretary of State's office as of the Effective Date.

ARTICLE III
FEES AND EXPENSE REIMBURSEMENT

Section 3.1. Professional Services.

(a) DEF will pay ABC fees for the SPECIALTY Services at the rate set forth below per Work Relative Value Unit ("**wRVU**"). Notwithstanding any future change made by the Centers for Medicare & Medicaid Services ("**CMS**") throughout the Term, or unless otherwise agreed by the parties during the

Checkpoint Period, the wRVUs generated by the Physicians in each Contract Year will be tabulated based on the weight assigned to each Common Procedural Terminology ("**CPT**") code by CMS in 2016, after being appropriately adjusted for modifiers. For purposes of this Agreement, "**Contract Year**" shall mean each twelve month period that this Agreement is in effect beginning on the Effective Date for the first Contract Year and the anniversary thereof for each subsequent Contract Year. All legitimate encounters will be recognized for their wRVU values regardless of the payer (or charity care) status of the patient. Compensation will be determined based on wRVU production of individual Physicians; however, the total compensation will be paid to ABC and not to the individual Physicians or specialties. The wRVU rates for Contract Years one (1) through three (3) are as follows:

	Rates per wRVU		
	Contract Year One	**Contract Year Two**	**Contract Year Three**
ABC	$67	$67	$67

Notwithstanding the foregoing, for the first three Contract Years, and for Contract Years four and five subject to any modifications agreed to by the parties pursuant to Section 3.1(c) or 4.2(b), DEF shall provide a minimum income guarantee (the "**Minimum Income Guarantee**") to ABC based on ABC's average total compensation of the last two (2) years prior to the Effective Date. The Minimum Income Guarantee shall be equal to ninety percent (90%) of the sum of each Physicians' W-2 income plus retirement contributions, health benefits, and other pre-tax benefits paid by ABC from the most recent two (2) full fiscal years less the other income that will be retained by ABC. The Minimum Income Guarantee shall be adjusted proportionally, at the individual Physician level, for changes in full time equivalent status. Payment to ABC of the full amount of the Minimum Income Guarantee will require the Physicians to maintain wRVU production greater than or equal to ninety percent (90%) of their historical levels based on an average of the Physicians' last two (2) years' average production (the "**Threshold**"), and if the Threshold is not met, the Minimum Income Guarantee will be adjusted by the same percentage by which the Threshold is not met; *provided* that in no event will the adjustment reduce the Minimum Income Guarantee by more ten percent (10%). By way of example, if the Physicians' wRVU production equals eighty-nine percent (89%) of their historical levels based on an average of the Physicians' last two (2) years' average production, the Minimum Income Guarantee shall be changed to eighty-nine percent (89%) of such historical levels.

(b) DEF shall pay ABC monthly draw payments equal to 90% of the prior year's production-based compensation for each Physician. At the end of each quarter, DEF shall determine the compensation payable to ABC for that period pursuant to Section 3.1(a). If the production-based compensation exceeds the sum of the draw payments paid to ABC, then the difference shall be paid to ABC by DEF within forty-five (45) days of the end of the quarter. If the sum of the draw payments paid to ABC for the period exceeds the production based compensation, then the difference shall be paid to DEF by ABC within forty-five (45) days of the end of the quarter.

(c) Prior to the end of the eighth (8th) month of the third Contract Year, DEF shall have obtained from a reputable valuation company reasonably acceptable to ABC a valuation of compensation for the fourth and fifth Contract Years. DEF shall inform ABC of the wRVU rate that shall apply for the fourth and fifth Contract Years, which shall be consistent with such valuation and in no event less than the wRVU rate for the third Contract Year, no later than the end of the eighth (8th) month of the third Contract Year. If such compensation is not acceptable to ABC, ABC will have the right to give notice of termination of this Agreement at least ninety (90) days prior to the end of the third Contract Year, to be effective at the end of the third Contract Year. This process shall be repeated during subsequent Contract Years when compensation may be adjusted for the following year so that ABC is given one month to decide whether to give ninety (90) days' notice of termination or to accept the revised compensation for the following year; *provided, however,* that for purposes of the Initial Term, if ABC does not exercise its right to terminate prior to the end of the third Contract Year, ABC shall have no further termination right pursuant to this Section 3.1(c) until after the end of the fifth Contract Year.

(d) If the parties determine during the Checkpoint Period (as defined in Section 4.2(b)) that, assuming consistent volumes, professional services reimbursement from all sources (including Medicare, Medicaid, and all private payers) in total has declined as of the 24th month of the Agreement by more than ten percent (10%) in comparison to reimbursement as of the 12th month of the Agreement, then DEF may propose to ABC, no later than the end of the tenth (10th) month of the third Contract Year, an adjusted compensation structure for the fourth and fifth Contract Years. If such adjusted compensation structure is not acceptable to ABC, ABC will have the right to give notice of termination of this Agreement pursuant to Section 4.2(b). In no event will the compensation be adjusted in the first three (3) Contract Years.

Other Payment Arrangements. The parties acknowledge that additional payment terms will be set forth in the other Transaction Agreements.

Reporting. On a monthly basis, DEF shall provide reports to ABC regarding financial and operational performance of the SPECIALTY Services, including without limitation volumes of procedures, expenses, wRVU rates, encounters and other data relevant to the SPECIALTY Services, all in a form and format acceptable to ABC. During the Term and for a two (2) year period after the termination of this Agreement, DEF shall provide ABC with access upon request to DEF's books and records for purposes of reviewing, verifying and calculating the compensation paid to ABC as described herein.

ARTICLE IV
TERM OF AGREEMENT

Section 4.1. Term. The initial term of this Agreement shall be for a period of five (5) years, commencing on the Effective Date (the "**Initial Term**"). The Agreement will automatically extend for consecutive five (5) year extension term(s) ("**Extension Terms**") upon the expiration of the Initial Term or applicable Extension Terms unless either party gives the other party written notice of its intent not to extend the Agreement no later than six (6) months prior to the expiration of the Initial Term or the applicable Extension Term. The Initial Term and each Extension Term may be referred to collectively as the "**Term**."

Section 4.2. Termination.

(a) Either party may terminate this Agreement by providing the other party with thirty (30) days' advance written notice if the PSSA is terminated.

(b) During the 4th through 9th months of the third Contract Year (the "**Checkpoint Period**"), the parties will review applicable data generated from the first two years of the Initial Term. At the end of the Checkpoint Period, either party may provide thirty (30) days' written notice to terminate this Agreement, with such termination to be effective on the last day of the third Contract Year. Additionally, during the Checkpoint Period, or at such other time throughout the Term of this Agreement, the parties will enter into good faith negotiations to specifically assess whether an employment option (such as, but not limited to, an arrangement in which the physicians are employed by DEF but retain, through ABC, ownership of the practice assets and employment of the non-physician practice personnel) is more desirable, and will consider regulatory and other market changes.

(c) This Agreement may also be terminated as set forth in Sections 4.3 and 4.4.

(d) In the event of a termination pursuant to this Section 4.2 or Sections 4.3 or 4.4, ABC will have the option to purchase all assets acquired by DEF from ABC in connection with this Agreement and the Transaction Agreements at the then fair market value. The fair market value of such assets, for purposes of such purchase, shall be determined by a mutually acceptable valuation company at the time of such purchase.

Section 4.3. Termination by ABC. ABC may terminate this Agreement prior to the end of a Term upon the occurrence of any one or more of the following by providing written notice to DEF or GHI:

(a) If DEF or GHI shall default in the performance of any material covenant, agreement, term or provision of this Agreement, or any other of the Transaction Agreements, and such default shall continue for a period of thirty (30) days after written notice to DEF or GHI from ABC stating the specific default (unless DEF or GHI commences to diligently pursue correction if such default is of a nature that cannot be reasonably corrected within said thirty (30) day period);

(b) If the DEF facilities necessary to provide the SPECIALTY Services or any portion thereof shall be damaged or destroyed, or if any of the SPECIALTY Services shall be rendered incapable of normal operation, by fire or other casualty, and if DEF fails to commence repairing, restoring, rebuilding or replacing any such damage or destruction within thirty (30) days after such fire or other casualty, or fails to complete such work within a reasonable period of time; provided, however, that DEF shall be under no obligation to repair, restore, rebuild, or replace any facility that is subject to a lease agreement between DEF and ABC or an affiliate of either party;

(c) If DEF or GHI shall apply for or consent to the appointment of a receiver, trustee or liquidator of DEF or GHI or of all or a substantial part of their assets, file a voluntary petition in bankruptcy or admit in writing its inability to pay its debts as they come due, make a general assignment for the benefit of creditors, file a petition or an answer seeking reorganization or arrangement with creditors of DEF or GHI, or file an involuntary petition under any state or federal reorganization, insolvency, arrangement, bankruptcy or other debtor relief provision, and such petition is not dismissed within thirty (30) days;

(d) If, through no fault of ABC, any license necessary for the operation of the Hospital or its SPECIALTY Services, or both, is at any time suspended, terminated or revoked; or

(e) If DEF or GHI shall fail to make payment to ABC when such payment becomes due and payable hereunder and does not make such payment within thirty (30) days after receiving written notice of such failure from ABC.

Section 4.4. Termination by DEF or GHI. DEF or GHI may terminate this Agreement prior to the end of a Term upon the occurrence of any one or more of the following by providing written notice to ABC:

(a) If ABC shall default in the performance of any material covenant, agreement, term or provision of this Agreement, or any other of the Transaction Agreements, and such default shall continue for a period of thirty (30) days after written notice to ABC from DEF or GHI stating the specific default (unless ABC begins to diligently pursue correction if such default is of a nature that cannot be reasonably corrected within said thirty (30) day period); or

(b) If ABC shall apply for or consent to the appointment of a receiver, trustee, or liquidator of ABC or of all or a substantial part of its assets, file a voluntary petition in bankruptcy, admit in writing its inability to pay its debts as they come due, make general assignment for the benefit of creditors, file a petition or an answer seeking reorganization or arrangement with creditors of ABC in an involuntary petition under any state or federal reorganization, insolvency, arrangement, bankruptcy or other debtor relief provision, and such petition is not dismissed within thirty (30) days.

Section 4.5. Obligations Upon Termination.

(a) In the event of any termination under the terms of this Agreement, each party shall cooperate with and assist the other party in the orderly and efficient transfer of all services to a successor or successors, as requested, prior to the termination date.

(b) Each party shall return to the other party any equipment or other items in its possession owned by the other party.

(c) The parties acknowledge and agree that, in the event this Agreement is terminated for any reason during the first twelve (12) months of the Initial Term, they shall not enter into an arrangement that is the same or substantially similar to the arrangement set forth in this Agreement for the balance of such twelve (12) month period.

(d) Upon termination of this Agreement, neither party shall have any further obligation hereunder except for (i) obligations accruing prior to the date of termination and (ii) obligations, promises, or covenants contained herein which are expressly made to extend beyond the Term of this Agreement, including, without limitation, any indemnification and insurance obligations.

ARTICLE V
LIABILITIES AND INSURANCE

Section 5.1. Indemnification by DEF and GHI. DEF and GHI shall jointly and severally indemnify and hold harmless ABC and its officers, agents and employees from any loss, cost, damage, expense, attorneys' fees and liability by reason of personal injury or property damage of whatsoever nature or kind, arising out of or as a result of the sole negligent act or failure to act of DEF or GHI or any of their employees or agents (other than ABC). This indemnification shall not apply if and to the extent the existence of this indemnification obligation restricts the application of professional liability insurance coverage to DEF or GHI or any of their employees pursuant to the provisions of any such policy.

Section 5.2. Indemnification by ABC. ABC shall indemnify and hold harmless DEF and GHI and their officers, agents and employees from any loss, cost, damage, expense, attorneys' fees and liability by reason of personal injury or property damage of whatsoever nature or kind, arising out of or as a result of the sole negligent act or failure to act of ABC or its employees or agents. This indemnification shall not apply if and to the extent the existence of this indemnification obligation restricts the application of professional liability insurance coverage to ABC or any of its physician employees pursuant to the provisions of any such policy.

Section 5.3. ABC Insurance. ABC shall, at its sole cost and expense, procure, keep and maintain throughout the Term of this Agreement, insurance coverage in the minimum amounts of: One Million Dollars ($1,000,000) per occurrence and Two Million Dollars ($2,000,000) annual aggregate for commercial general liability. Throughout the Term of this Agreement, ABC shall maintain professional liability insurance for its physicians with limits of not less than One Million Dollars ($1,000,000) per claim and Three Million Dollars ($3,000,000) in the aggregate, workers' compensation insurance and other mandatory statutory insurance relating to its employees. DEF shall reimburse ABC for its costs of providing professional liability insurance for its physicians as set forth in other Transaction Agreements. Upon termination of this Agreement, ABC shall continue the insurance coverage for its physicians, in the amounts stated above, with a non-advancing retroactive date or purchase tail coverage for professional malpractice alleged to have occurred during the Term of this Agreement, as applicable. ABC shall give

DEF evidence of the foregoing insurance before rendering services hereunder and on an annual basis thereafter. ABC shall immediately notify DEF, in writing, of any termination, cancellation or reduction of such coverage or any failure to renew such coverage during the Term of this Agreement.

Section 5.4. GHI Insurance. GHI shall, at its sole cost and expense, procure, keep and maintain throughout the Term of this Agreement, insurance coverage in the minimum amounts of One Million Dollars ($1,000,000) per occurrence and Three Million Dollars ($3,000,000) annual aggregate for professional liability and One Million Dollars ($1,000,000) per occurrence and Two Million Dollars ($2,000,000) annual aggregate for commercial general liability. GHI shall also maintain in full force and effect all required workers' compensation mandated by the State of STATE, as applicable. GHI may meet its obligations under this Section 5.4 through self- insurance or a captive insurance company.

ARTICLE VI
CONFIDENTIALITY; OWNERSHIP OF MEDICAL RECORDS

Section 6.1. Confidentiality. Each party acknowledges that it will receive proprietary data and confidential information regarding the practices of the other party and its affiliates. Such data and information include, without limitation, costs, profits, patient names and medical records and any other confidential data or information, whether or not of a similar nature (the "**Information**"). Each party acknowledges that its relationship to the other party and its affiliates with respect to the other party's Information is fiduciary in nature and that it shall not make use of such Information except in the discharge of its obligations hereunder. Each party shall maintain the terms of this Agreement and the Information in the strictest of confidence and in full compliance with applicable laws and regulations.

Section 6.2. Ownership of Medical Records. Patients receiving services hereunder are patients of DEF. All medical records of such patients shall be and remain the property of DEF and shall not be removed or transferred from DEF except in accordance with applicable state and federal laws and regulations and in conformity with DEF's bylaws, rules, regulations, policies and procedures. ABC shall have access to such medical records during and after the Term of this Agreement as requested by ABC or a ABC patient and as permitted by law. Notwithstanding the foregoing, following termination of this Agreement, the non-provider based medical records shall be maintained by ABC, and DEF shall have access to these medical records following the Term hereof as permitted by law.

ARTICLE VII
GOVERNANCE AND EXCLUSIVITY

Section 7.1. ABC Retained Powers. During the Term, ABC will remain as an independent for-profit medical practice. The Physicians and support staff will remain governed by ABC's by-laws, policies and procedures. Without limiting the generality of the foregoing, ABC will continue to have full control over the following activities, subject to DEF's reserved powers as the sole member of GHI:

   (a) Group governance
   (b) Physician hiring and termination
   (c) Income distribution
   (d) Clinical practice and quality control
   (e) Malpractice coverage
   (f) Staffing and personnel management
   (g) Computer technology and information system
   (h) Non-ancillary assets
   (i) Operating and capital budgets

Section 7.2. DEF Retained Control. DEF shall at all times exercise control over the assets and operation of DEF. By entering into this Agreement, DEF does not delegate to ABC any of the powers, duties and responsibilities required to be retained by DEF under law (including all certificates and licenses issued under authority of law for SPECIALTY Services). DEF shall be the holder of all licenses, accreditation certificates and contracts that DEF obtains and shall be the technical or facility "provider" within the meaning of all third-party contracts for the SPECIALTY Services.

Section 7.3. PSA Executive Committee. To achieve value-exchange goals, DEF and ABC will jointly establish a committee (the "**Executive Committee**") to oversee certain joint governance matters. The Executive Committee will consist of three (3) ABC members elected by the ABC's executive committee ("**ABC Members**"), and two (2) members selected by the DEF's administrative leadership team ("**DEF Members**"). Primary duties of the Executive Committee are to jointly develop strategic plans relative to the service line and the operations of this Agreement. The Executive Committee will collect recommendations from ABC and DEF and meet on a monthly basis. A quorum shall exist at a meeting of the Executive Committee if at least two (2) ABC Members and one (1) DEF Member are present at the meeting. During the monthly meetings, the Executive Committee will discuss and vote on matters that have been recommended to the Executive Committee. For purposes of taking action at a meeting of the Executive Committee, ABC and DEF shall each have one (1) vote, and ABC and DEF shall each act through their ABC Members and DEF members, respectively. The ABC Members and the DEF Members in attendance at a meeting of the Executive Committee at which quorum exists must reach consensus among themselves on how to cast their one (1) vote. The approval or consent of both ABC and DEF at a meeting at which a quorum exists shall be required for the Executive Committee to take action.

Section 7.4. Income Distribution Plan. ABC will be solely responsible for the creation and implementation of an income distribution plan with respect to the ABC providers. ABC will annually provide to DEF a certification from a duly-appointed officer of ABC that ABC's income distribution plan is in compliance with all applicable laws and regulations.

Section 7.5. Collaboration on Reimbursement Initiatives. Before undertaking any new reimbursement initiatives such as bundled payments, the parties will discuss and agree upon each party's role with respect to the new reimbursement arrangements and whether adjustments to the fees payable under this Agreement or any Transaction Agreement are necessary or appropriate in light of the new arrangements.

Section 7.6. Technology.

(a) If ABC, at the sole request of DEF, implements a new technology system (e.g. email, EHR, etc.), DEF will bear 100% of the upfront, interface development and implementation costs associated with the new technology. DEF will also be responsible for any costs associated with the termination of existing contracts ABC holds with their current technology vendors. ABC will have access to patient electronic health records and practice management information from the new technology systems for a period of up to two (2) years after termination of this Agreement. DEF will be responsible for any costs associated with the interface or modification of current ABC systems to meet DEF system requirements.

Section 7.7. Noncompetition. During the Term of this Agreement and for a period of one (1) year following the effective date of termination of this Agreement (the "**Noncompetition Period**"), ABC and the Physicians shall not within ten (10) miles of any DEF facility (the "**Restricted Area**") directly or indirectly hold an ownership interest in, serve as an officer or director of, be employed by, or render services or advice to, any corporation, partnership, limited liability company, proprietorship or other business enterprise that provides, contracts for the provision of, or holds itself out to the public as a provider of, professional medical services, including SPECIALTY services or interventional procedures performed in a SPECIALTY laboratory, and is (i) a hospital or health system that competes with DEF or an affiliate of DEF (an "**Institution**"); (ii) any other business enterprise that controls, is controlled by, or is under common control with an Institution; or (iii) an Institution that is located outside of the Restricted Area and provides services within the Restricted Area; provided, however, that nothing in this Section 7.7 shall prohibit ABC or any Physician from (x) providing professional services to patients at an Institution, or (y) entering into an employment or other relationship with a physician organization that operates no impatient facility. During the Term of this Agreement, ABC shall cause the Physicians to collectively provide services on a full-time basis in accordance with Section 1.2(b). Notwithstanding the foregoing, ABC or a Physician may continue to hold an ownership interest in a competing Institution if ABC or the Physician acquired such ownership interest prior to the Effective Date of this Agreement. The provision of services other than SPECIALTY Services and the provision of Excluded Services shall not be considered being in competition with DEF for this purpose. Notwithstanding the foregoing, this covenant shall not prevent ABC from referring to, or providing clinical services at, other facilities (other than pursuant to a services arrangement as described above). In addition, this covenant shall not prevent ABC, following termination of this Agreement, from operating as an independent physician practice.

Section 7.8. Services & Locations. Expansion of DEF's SPECIALTY-related services (specifically including SPECIALTY rehabilitation) will be located at ABC's main office location on Gaslight Boulevard. Specifically, pursuant to the New Programs Lease, all available space on the second floor of the main office will be leased to DEF for purposes of the expanded SPECIALTY-related services. Throughout the Term, Physicians and any other ABC providers may practice medicine at non-DEF-affiliated facilities, including Woodland Heights Medical Center. ABC will continue to perform the SPECIALTY Services currently provided by ABC throughout the Term of the Agreement.

Section 7.9. Added Services & Locations. The parties will use their reasonable best efforts to develop additional clinical services within the DEF service area and to expand the geographical outreach for DEF clinical services. ABC shall have a right of first refusal to provide all professional services for any such functional or geographic expansion of services.

Section 7.10. Reasonable Time for Staffing and Training. The Executive Committee shall, in consultation with DEF and ABC, identify needs for additional physicians and other staff or for training in new modalities and techniques. Once such need is agreed to by the Executive Committee, ABC will use its reasonable best efforts to add such necessary physicians and staff, or to provide adequate training in new modalities and techniques to existing physicians and staff, within twelve (12) months. If ABC is not able to do so or elects not to do so within twelve (12) months, the affected DEF facility will be permitted to retain other professionals to provide such services.

Section 7.11. Recruiting. DEF and ABC, through the Executive Committee, shall discuss and mutually agree upon whether and when additional physicians are recruited and what specialties and/or other recruiting qualifications are necessary to meet the needs of the pertinent service line(s) and the communities served by DEF and the ABC facilities. The process will be completed in accordance with the findings of DEF's then-current community needs assessment which will quantify the need for additional providers to the community.

(a) If the Executive Committee determines there is a need for one (1) or more additional physicians, ABC shall have thirty (30) days to determine whether it will recruit one (1) or more of the additional physicians into its practice; provided, however, that once two (2) new physicians have been added to ABC, DEF shall have the right of first election on the third recruit.

(i) If ABC elects to recruit additional physicians, it shall notify DEF of its intention within thirty (30) days after the Executive Committee's decision to recruit. ABC shall then proceed to recruit for the position with the administrative and financial support of DEF as provided below in Section 7.11(c). When ABC has identified a candidate (a "**Candidate**"), DEF shall have the right to accept or reject the identified Candidate for good cause based on professional qualifications, or such other good cause as shall be clearly demonstrated. DEF's approval of ABC's decision to recruit a Candidate shall not be unreasonably withheld. In the event DEF rejects the Candidate, ABC recruiting will recommence.

(ii) If ABC elects not to recruit additional physicians, it shall notify DEF of its decision not to recruit within thirty (30) days after the Executive Committee's decision to recruit, and DEF may elect to recruit.

(b) If the Executive Committee cannot reach a consensus concerning the need for additional physicians, and either ABC or DEF deems recruitment necessary and supported by community need as demonstrated by the then-current DEF community needs assessment, the dispute shall be resolved in the manner described in Article 9 ("Dispute Resolution") of the PSSA through mediation and failing resolution, binding arbitration.

(c) DEF shall bear reasonable administrative costs associated with recruiting additional physicians once the Executive Committee has agreed on the need for recruiting, and shall provide such administrative support as shall be reasonably necessary to facilitate the recruiting. Costs of recruiting may include, without limitation, recruiting or finder's fees, and reasonable costs associated with investigation and interview of potential candidate(s) as the parties shall agree. Subject to demonstration of community need, DEF will provide appropriate recruitment incentives and income support (e.g., signing bonus, relocation expenses, income guarantee or other support) as shall be mutually agreed by the parties and in compliance with applicable law.

(d) DEF shall not, without the consent of ABC, enter into an employment relationship with any SPECIALIST practicing within the Restricted Area as of the Effective Date.

Section 7.12. Attrition Protection. During the Term and pursuant to the terms of this Section 7.12, GHI will protect ABC from a decrease in the average individual ABC Physician's wRVU production that results from the addition of new physicians to ABC or DEF ("**Attrition**"). If (i) the average wRVU production per-FTE ABC Physician for a Contract Year ("**Average wRVU Production**") is less than the average wRVU production per-FTE ABC Physician based on the most recent two years preceding the applicable Contract Year ("**Baseline wRVU Production**") (the difference between the Average wRVU Production and the Baseline wRVU Production shall be considered the "**wRVU Deficiency**") and (ii) such wRVU Deficiency is found to have been caused by Attrition, then ABC's total wRVU production for that Contract Year shall be adjusted in accordance with the following procedure:

(a) If ABC believes that a wRVU Deficiency during a Contract Year was caused by Attrition, then, within thirty (30) days following the end of that Contract Year, ABC shall deliver notice to the Executive Committee setting forth the specific reasons that ABC believes the wRVU Deficiency is related to Attrition, such as the hiring of additional physicians.

(b) Immediately upon notice under Section 7.12(a), the Executive Committee shall determine whether the wRVU Deficiency primarily was caused by Attrition. In making such determination, the Executive Committee shall take into account the collective work effort of the ABC Physicians, as measured by factors such as availability to provide professional services to patients. In the event that the Executive Committee determines that the collective ABC level of work effort has declined substantially, in the absence of other factors, the ABC Members or DEF Members of the Executive Committee shall not unreasonably withhold a vote that the wRVU Deficiency primarily was caused by Attrition. The Executive Committee's recommendation shall be binding unless contrary to law or ethics.

(c) ABC's total wRVU production for a Contract Year shall be adjusted by adding seventy-five percent (75%) of the wRVU Deficiency in the first Contract Year following the addition of a new physician and, if the wRVU Deficiency is found to have continued into a second year, then fifty percent (50%) of the wRVU Deficiency shall be added to ABC's total wRVU production in the second Contract Year after the addition of a new physician.

(d) GHI shall pay the additional compensation computed under this methodology within ninety (90) days following the end of a Contract Year.

Section 7.13. Replacement Physicians. Upon termination or retirement of a ABC Physician or physician employed by DEF, if there is a need for a replacement, ABC (in the case of a replacement of a formerly ABC-employed Physician), or DEF (in the case of a replacement of a formerly DEF-employed physician), will supply such replacement as quickly as practicable, unless otherwise decided by the Executive Committee through the process described in Section 7.3. The selection of the replacement physician will be in the sole discretion of ABC or DEF, as applicable, but each of ABC and DEF will agree to consult with one another regarding professional and personal qualifications of the replacement before he or she is hired. DEF will provide appropriate recruitment assistance and incentives (e.g., signing bonus, moving expenses, income guarantees) as mutually agreed by the parties and in compliance with applicable law.

ARTICLE VIII
MISCELLANEOUS

Section 8.1. Representations and Warranties of the Parties. Each party represents and warrants to the other parties hereto that:

(a) Such party is duly organized, validly existing and in good standing under the laws of the State of STATE with qualification to do business in the State of STATE.

(b) Such party is authorized to enter into this Agreement by all necessary and proper action, and this Agreement has been duly and validly executed and delivered by such party and is a legal, valid and binding agreement of such party, enforceable against it in accordance with its terms.

Section 8.2. Compliance with All Laws, Regulations and Standards.

(a) **Compliance with Laws.** Each party shall comply with all applicable federal, state and local statutes, rules and regulations, and it shall be deemed a material breach of this Agreement if a party shall fail to comply with this requirement.

(b) **Confidentiality of Patient Information.** Each party shall protect the confidentiality of any patient's clinical and private information, and shall comply with all laws applicable to the confidentiality of patient information. Each party is a Covered Entity as defined by the Administrative Simplification requirements of the Health Insurance Portability and Accountability Act of 1996 ("**HIPAA**") and regulations promulgated thereunder, including the Standards for Privacy of Individually Identifiable Health Information and Security Standards for the Protection of Electronic Protected Health Information at 45 C.F.R. Parts 160 and 164, as such standards are amended from time to time, including, without limitation, the amendments to such standards contained in the American Recovery and Reinvestment Act of 2009 (the "**Privacy and Security Regulations**"). To the extent that either party is acting as a Business Associate (as defined by HIPAA) of the other party with respect to the services to be provided pursuant to this Agreement or any Transaction Agreement, the parties agrees to comply with the requirements set forth in *Exhibit 8.2* to this Agreement.

(c) **Survival.** This Section shall survive the termination of this Agreement.

Section 8.3. Exclusion from Medicare or Medicaid. Each party hereby represents and warrants that such party, its members, agents or employees are not and at no time have been excluded from participation in any federally funded health care program, including Medicare and Medicaid. Each party hereby agrees to immediately notify the other party of any threatened, proposed or actual exclusion of such party, its members, agents or employees from any federally funded health care program, including Medicare and Medicaid. In the event that a party, or any of its members, agents or employees are excluded from participation in any federally funded health care program during the term of this Agreement, or if at any time after the Effective Date it is determined that a party is in breach of the requirements contained in this Section, the other party shall have the right to immediately terminate this Agreement as of the effective date of such exclusion or breach. Notwithstanding the foregoing, in the event that a person employed by a party is excluded from participation in any federally funded health care program, such party may remedy the exclusion from Medicare or Medicaid by terminating such person from employment and by promptly providing a replacement acceptable to the other party to provide any services to have been provided hereunder by the excluded person.

Section 8.4. Dispute Resolution Procedure. Any dispute or claim arising out of or relating to this Agreement, or a breach hereof, shall be resolved in accordance with this Section 8.4. During the course of resolving any such dispute, ABC shall continue to perform its obligations and otherwise abide by the requirements under this Agreement. Notwithstanding the foregoing, the obligation of ABC to continue to perform hereunder during the resolution of disputes shall not require GHI to perform obligations where such performance is rendered impossible, or would otherwise not maintain or increase the likelihood that GHI will achieve its business purpose, because of circumstances created by or directly related to the dispute itself.

(a) **Good Faith Consultation.** In the event of a dispute between the parties, representatives of the parties shall attempt in good faith to settle such dispute through mutual consultation. If, after such consultation, the dispute cannot be resolved, the parties' representatives shall wait for not less than thirty (30) days after the dispute arises and at the end of such period meet for a second consultation; *provided* that such period shall be shortened in the event the parties' representatives agree that the dispute, or the results, thereof, will only become more intractable or cause more damage with the passage of time. If the dispute is not resolved after the second consultation, the matter shall be referred to the Executive Committee. If the Executive Committee is unable to resolve the dispute within sixty (60) days after the second consultation, then the dispute shall be referred to mediation.

(b) **Mediation.** If a dispute arises relating to this Agreement and cannot be resolved through the good faith consultation process set forth above, then the parties will first proceed in good faith to submit the matter to mediation. Either party may request mediation by notifying the other party in writing of its desire to submit the matter to mediation. Within ten (10) business days following notice of intent to proceed to mediation, the parties shall jointly select, appoint and arrange to meet with an impartial person who can mediate and facilitate the parties toward a resolution using an informal and confidential process. The mediator cannot impose binding decisions on the parties. The parties must agree to the terms of any settlement arising out of the mediation process in order for such agreement to become binding. The parties will share equally in the cost of such mediation, regardless of the outcome of the process. The mediation, unless otherwise agreed, shall terminate if the parties have not been able to resolve the dispute within thirty (30) calendar days from the date when mediation meetings began. Upon such termination, either party may pursue the arbitration process set forth in Section 8.4(c).

(c) **Arbitration.** Any arbitration to be conducted hereunder shall be brought and conducted in accordance with the following provisions.

(i) The parties agree to refer such dispute to binding arbitration to a single Arbitrator selected by the American Health Lawyers Association. Such referral shall be made within sixty (60) days of the last attempted resolution by the parties.

(ii) The arbitration shall be governed by the current rules and procedures of the American Health Lawyers Association to the extent that such rules are not inconsistent with this Agreement. The compensation and expenses of the Arbitrator and any administrative fees or costs associated with the arbitration proceedings shall be borne equally by the parties.

(iii) The decision of the Arbitrator(s) shall be final, conclusive, and binding, and no action at law or in equity may be instituted by either party other than to enforce the award of the Arbitrator(s).

(iv) Arbitration proceedings shall take place in the State of STATE.

Section 8.5. Notices. Except as provided otherwise in this Agreement, any and all notices necessary or desirable to be served hereunder shall be in writing and shall be delivered personally, sent by certified mail or overnight delivery service to the intended recipient at the address for such intended recipient set forth below, or sent by facsimile to the fax number for such intended recipient set forth below, or to such other address or facsimile number as the party may designate in writing.

If to GHI: GHI Clinical Services
1234 Main Street
CITY, STATE 00000
Attention: Mr. John Doe

If to DEF: DEF Hospital
1234 Main Street
CITY, STATE 00000
Attention: Mr. John Doe

If to ABC: ABC Specialty Practice, P.A.
             123 Elm Street
             CITY, STATE 00000
             Attention: John Doe, M.D.

Any notice sent by mail as provided above shall be deemed delivered on the second (2nd) business day following the postmark date which it bears. Any notice sent by facsimile or hand delivery as provided above shall be deemed delivered when sent. Any notice sent by a nationally recognized overnight carrier shall be deemed delivered on the next business day following the postmarked date which it bears.

Section 8.6. Assignment. Neither party shall have the right to assign its rights or delegate its duties hereunder to any party unless it first obtains the written consent of the other party, which party may grant or deny in its sole and absolute discretion.

Section 8.7. Successors and Assigns. This Agreement and the rights, privileges, duties and obligations of the parties hereunder, to the extent assignable or delegable, shall be binding upon and inure to the benefit of the parties and their respective successors and permitted assignees.

Section 8.8. Amendments. This Agreement may be amended at any time by mutual agreement of the parties without additional consideration, provided that before any amendment shall become effective, it shall be reduced to writing and signed by each of the parties.

Section 8.9. Governing Law. This Agreement shall be governed by and construed in accordance with the laws of the State of STATE applicable to agreements made and to be performed wholly within that state, irrespective of such state's choice-of-law principles.

Section 8.10. Integration. This Agreement, along with its exhibits, which are hereby incorporated by reference, constitutes the entire agreement between the parties with respect to its subject matter. The parties acknowledge that they are, simultaneously with this Agreement, entering into the Transaction Agreements.

Section 8.11. Severability. If any term of this Agreement shall to any extent be invalid and unenforceable, the remainder of this Agreement shall not be affected thereby, and each term of this Agreement shall be enforced to the extent permitted by law.

Section 8.12. Waiver. All waivers of rights, powers and remedies by a party to this Agreement must be in writing. No delay, omission or failure by a party to exercise any right, power or remedy to which a party may be entitled shall impair any such right, power or remedy, nor shall such be construed as a release by a party of such right, power or remedy or as a waiver of or acquiescence in any such action, unless such action shall have been cured in accordance with the terms of this Agreement. A waiver by a party of any right, power or remedy in any one instance shall not constitute a waiver of the same or any other right, power or remedy in any other instance.

Section 8.13. Medicare Access to Books and Records. If and to the extent required by Section 1395x(v)(1)(I) of Title 42 of the United States Code, until the expiration of four (4) years after the termination of this Agreement, each party shall make available, upon written request by the Secretary of the Department of Health and Human Services, or upon request by the Comptroller General of the United States General Accounting Office, or any of their duly authorized representatives, a copy of this Agreement and such books, documents and records as are necessary to certify the nature and extent of the costs of the services provided by such party under this Agreement. Each party further agrees that in the event such party carries out any of its duties under this Agreement through a subcontract with a related organization with a value or cost of Ten Thousand Dollars ($10,000.00) or more over a twelve (12) month period, such subcontract shall contain a provision requiring the related organization to make available until the expiration of four (4) years after the furnishing of such services pursuant to such subcontract upon written request to the Secretary of the United States Department of Health and Human Services, or upon request to the Comptroller General of the United States General Accounting Office, or any of their duly authorized representatives, a copy of such subcontract and such books, documents and records of such organization as are necessary to verify the nature and extent of such costs.

Section 8.14. No Third-Party Rights. This Agreement has been made and is made solely for the benefit of the parties hereto and their respective successors and permitted assigns. Nothing in this Agreement is intended to confer any rights or remedies under or by reason of this Agreement on any persons other than the parties to it and their respective successors and permitted assigns. Nothing in this Agreement is intended to relieve or discharge the obligation or liability of any third persons to any party to this Agreement.

Section 8.15. Headings. The subject headings of the sections and paragraphs of this Agreement are included for purposes of convenience only and shall not affect the construction or interpretation of any of its provisions. Throughout this Agreement, the singular shall include the plural, the plural shall include the singular, and the masculine and neuter shall include the feminine, wherever the context so requires.

Section 8.16. Compliance. The parties agree that nothing contained in this Agreement shall require ABC to refer or admit patients to, or order any goods or services from, DEF or any other DEF entity. Notwithstanding any unanticipated effect of any provision of this Agreement, neither party will knowingly or intentionally conduct its behavior in such a manner as to violate the prohibitions against fraud and abuse or self-referral prohibitions in connection with the Medicare and Medicaid programs. ABC physicians shall be free to join the medical staffs of other hospitals, and shall be entitled to refer patients to such hospitals.

Section 8.17. Electronic Disposition of Document (Scanning and Photocopies). The parties hereto agree and stipulate that the original of this document, including the signature page, may be scanned and stored in a computer database or similar device, and that any printout or other output readable by sight, the reproduction of which is shown to accurately reproduce the original of this document, may be used for any purpose just as if it were the original, including proof of the content of the original writing.

Section 8.18. Master List. DEF maintains a master list of contracts that is updated centrally and available for review by the Secretary of the Department of Health and Human Services upon request. The master list is maintained in a manner that preserves the historical records of contracts. The master list of contracts references all separate agreements among DEF, GHI, and ABC, or between DEF or GHI and any physician owners of ABC or their immediate family members (as defined in 42 C.F.R. § 411.351), in a manner that is intended to conform to the requirements of 42 C.F.R. § 411.357(d)(ii).

**** Remainder of Page Blank; Signature Page Follows ****

IN WITNESS WHEREOF, the parties hereto have executed this Agreement as of the day and year first above written.

GHI:

GHI Clinical Services

By: _____

Name: _____

Title: _____

ABC:

ABC Specialty Practice, P.A.

By: _____

Name: _____

Title: _____

DEF:

DEF Hospital

By: _____

Name: _____

Title: _____

APPENDIX D

MANAGEMENT AGREEMENT

THIS MANAGEMENT AGREEMENT (the "Agreement"), made and entered into as of the ____ day of MONTH YEAR ("Effective Date"), by and between **ABC HOSPITAL**, a STATE non-profit corporation (the "Client"); and **COKER GROUP HOLDINGS, LLC, dba COKER GROUP**, a Georgia limited liability company ("Coker").

WITNESSETH:

WHEREAS, Client desires to engage Coker, to provide an onsite consultant to fill the role of a POSITION and provide certain other general management consulting services in connection with the management and operation of certain physician employed networks that are owned by the Client (the "Business"), upon the conditions and terms herein set forth; and

WHEREAS, Coker desires to provide an onsite consultant to fill the role of POSITION and provide certain other general management consulting services in connection with the management and operation of Client's Business for and on behalf of Client, upon the terms and conditions hereinafter set forth;

NOW, THEREFORE, FOR AND IN CONSIDERATION of the mutual promises herein contained, and for other good and valuable consideration, the receipt, sufficiency and adequacy of which are hereby acknowledged, the parties hereto, each intending to be legally bound, do hereby agree as follows:

1. Engagement of Coker; Term; Termination Fee.

    (a) Client hereby engages Coker to provide general management consulting services in connection with the management and operation of Client's Business during the term of this Agreement, and Coker hereby accepts such engagement and agrees to perform the general management consulting services pursuant to the terms and conditions of this Agreement. Coker shall also provide an ACTING POSITION and a POSITION to Client pursuant to Section 3 of this Agreement.

    (b) This Agreement shall become effective as of the Effective Date and, unless sooner terminated pursuant to the provisions of this Agreement, shall remain in full force and effect for a period ending with the third anniversary of the Effective Date (the "Initial Term"). In the event neither party terminates this Agreement during the Initial Term then this Agreement shall automatically renew for a one year period upon each anniversary of the Effective Date ("Renewal Term") until terminated as provided for herein. The Initial Term and any Renewal Term(s) are sometimes hereinafter referred to as the "Term").

(c) Either party may terminate this Agreement for any reason whatsoever upon one hundred eighty (180) days' notice to the other party.

2. <u>Management Fee</u>.

(a) Coker shall be entitled to receive the following fees and expenses during the Initial Term of this Agreement payable as described in the table below. All fees due under this Section 2 are due and payable on the first day of each month except for expenses that are due to Coker within thirty days after receipt by Client of Coker's invoice containing expenses subject to reimbursement pursuant to this Agreement. At or prior to the end of the Initial Term of this Agreement, provided neither party has terminated this Agreement at or prior to the end of the Initial Term, the parties shall negotiate in good faith and mutually agree upon the management fees that Coker will be paid upon the beginning of the initial Renewal Term. The parties agree to negotiate in good faith and mutually agree upon the management fees that Coker will be paid upon the beginning any subsequent Renewal Term in the same manner as the parties did at or prior to the start of the initial Renewal Term.

Month	Payment	Purpose
Month 1 beginning on Execution date	$_____	General engagement fees
Month 2	$_____	General engagement fees
Month 3	$_____	General engagement fees
Month 4	$_____	General engagement fees
Month 5 and every month thereafter during the Term	$_____	General engagement fees
Month immediately after hiring of the POSITION and each month thereafter during the Term	See Section 2(b) and 2(c)	Base Salary, employee benefits (excluding bonus compensation) and expenses of POSITION

During the first four months of this Agreement or until the POSITION is hired and assumes his duties, whichever is sooner	See Section 2(d)	Expenses of ACTING POSITION
Month 5 and each month thereafter until the POSITION is hired	See Section 2(e)	Base Salary, employee benefits (excluding bonus compensation) and expenses of ACTING POSITION

(b) Coker shall provide a POSITION to Client pursuant to Section 3(b) of this Agreement. Client will be solely responsible for reimbursing Coker for the base salary and employee benefits (excluding bonus compensation that will be Coker's sole responsibility) that Coker pays to its employee who is performing the POSITION responsibilities for Client. Coker estimates that the salary in year one may be approximately $_____ and in year two such salary may be $_____. Coker estimates that employee benefits for the POSITION may cost between 20 and 25 percent of such employee's base salary. Coker and Client agree that the amounts stated here are estimates and the actual salary in year one or year two may be higher or lower than the estimate but in no event shall the base salary in either year exceed $_____. Coker and Client further agree that the employee benefits that Client is responsible for paying to Coker may be higher or lower than the estimate but in no event shall such benefits exceed 30 percent of the POSITION's base salary for the year in question. Coker agrees to provide Client reasonable documentation of the amount owed to Coker for such salary and employee benefits and Client shall pay such amount in equal installments (provided Coker may make reasonable adjustments to this amount to account for a 3 percent profit sharing contribution made by Coker on its employee's behalf or other employee benefits adjustments that Coker may make in the ordinary course of its business) payable on the first day of each month for the remainder of the Term of this Agreement with the first payment due on first day of the month immediately following the effective date of employment of the POSITION.

(c) Client agrees to reimburse Coker for the following expenses incurred in connection with the POSITION's performance of his duties pursuant to this Agreement:

  (i) Reasonable relocation expenses incurred in the POSITION moving to the area, including, without limitation, temporary housing for at least ninety (90) days and commuting expenses (including, without limitation, mileage, gasoline and car insurance) if the commute to Client's place of business is greater than 25 miles.

(ii) Membership dues in at least two professional organizations that the POSITION wishes to be a member.

(iii) Reimbursement for up to seven days per calendar year of workshops and conferences related to the performance of POSITION's duties hereunder or the healthcare industry and such reimbursement shall include, without limitation, workshop/conference fees, travel, meal and lodging expenses.

(iv) Professional development expenses, including, without, limitation, professional training.

(v) Business development and employee recruitment expenses, including, without limitation, business lunches and dinners and other entertainment of physician's or other prospective employees.

(vi) Ordinary and reasonable expenses incurred in the performance of the POSITION's duties hereunder.

(d) Upon the Effective Date of this Agreement, Coker shall provide an ACTING POSITION pursuant to Section 3(b) until a POSITION is hired and assumes his duties under this Agreement. During the first four months of this Agreement or until the hiring of the POSITION, whichever is sooner, Client shall not be responsible for reimbursing Coker for any base salary and employee benefits payable to the ACTING POSITION. Client shall only be responsible for paying the following expenses for the ACTING POSITION:

(i) Temporary housing for at least one hundred and twenty (120) days, including, without limitation, overnight stays at hotels or condominiums and associated meals while staying there.

(ii) Commuting expenses (including, without limitation, mileage, gasoline, car insurance and airfare).

(e) On the five-month anniversary of this Agreement, in the event that the POSITION has not been hired and assumed his duties under this Agreement, Client shall pay to Coker the following fees and expenses with respect to the ACTING POSITION each month during the Term of the Agreement until the POSITION begins employment with the Client:

(i) A monthly fee equal to $_____ that is derived by taking a salary of $_____ and multiplying such salary by 1.25 and then dividing the product of $_____ multiplied by 1.25 by 12 or ($_____ x 1.25 =$_____/12 =$_____ and rounded to $_____).

(ii) Temporary housing until the hiring of the POSITION, including, without limitation, overnight stays at hotels or condominiums and associated meals while staying there.

(iii) Commuting expenses (including, without limitation, mileage, gasoline car insurance and airfare).

(f) Coker and Client agree that the parties will negotiate in good faith to determine the criteria for awarding Coker an annual performance bonus for the services it performs pursuant to this Agreement no later than (90) days after the Effective Date of this Agreement. Such criteria shall also include the following: (1) the bonus shall be paid at least semiannually during each calendar year of this Agreement; and (2) Coker's eligibility for such bonus and how it is paid in the event of a termination of this Agreement by either party.

(g) Coker and Client agree that Coker has the right to request additional fees that the parties shall mutually agree upon in the event that the number of employed physician providers in the Business significantly increases. The parties agree to negotiate in good faith and agree upon such additional fees within thirty (30) days of Coker's written request for the additional fees along with a summary describing the facts giving rise to the additional fees. In general, Client currently has approximately _____ providers within the Business at the beginning of this Agreement. The Client anticipates significant growth during the contract term. Both Client and Coker agree to a $1,000 increase in the monthly fee for every ten (10) new providers. Should there be additional need, Coker and Client will continue to discuss and agree upon any additional increase to the monthly fee.

(h) In the event Client terminates this Agreement pursuant to Section 1(c) and Client gives such termination notice during the month described in the table below during the Initial Term of the Agreement, Client agrees to pay Coker, in addition to any fees due to Coker prior to the termination date of this Agreement under Section 1(c), a termination fee equal to the corresponding amount provided in the table below payable at the time Client gives Coker notice it wishes to terminate the Agreement pursuant to Section 1(c).

Month Termination Notice Given	Termination Fee
Any time prior to the 9-month anniversary of the Effective Date of this Agreement.	$_____
Nine months and one day from the Effective Date of this Agreement through and including the 12-month anniversary of the Effective Date of this Agreement.	$_____
Twelve months and one day from the Effective Date of this Agreement through the 18-month anniversary of the Effective Date of this Agreement.	$_____
Eighteen months and one day from the Effective Date of this Agreement through the 36-month anniversary of the Effective Date of this Agreement.	$_____

3. <u>Services of Coker</u>.

   (a) Coker shall be responsible for providing the services described on Exhibit "A" attached hereto and incorporated herein by this reference ("Duties and Responsibilities"). The ACTING POSITION or the POSITION (as defined in Section 3(b), as the case may be, has the absolute right to request and use additional Coker personnel to perform the Duties and Responsibilities required of Coker under the terms and conditions of this Agreement.

   (b) Upon execution of this Agreement Coker shall do the following:

   (i) Provide an employee of Coker, who shall be determined by Coker in its sole discretion, who shall act in the capacity of ACTING POSITION of the Client with respect to the Business and have the authority, in addition to Coker, to perform the services described in the Duties and Responsibilities Exhibit. The ACTING POSITION shall service until he is replaced by the POSITION pursuant to Section 3(b)(ii).

   (ii) Recruit and hire an employee of Coker, who shall be determined by Coker in its sole discretion, who shall act in the capacity of POSITION of the Client with respect to the Business who shall replace the ACTING POSITION and have the authority, in addition to Coker, to perform the services described in the Duties and Responsibilities Exhibit.

(c) Coker and Client agree that in the event the employment of the ACTING POSITION or the POSITION is terminated for any reason, the Client's sole remedy is to have Coker replace the ACTING POSITION or the POSITION, as the case may be, with a qualified replacement as determined by Coker, in its reasonable discretion, within thirty (30) days.

(d) Excluded Services: Coker and the Client agree that Coker is not providing to the Client the following specific services pursuant to this Agreement:

   (i) Valuation services for physician practices that become part of the Business.

   (ii) New information technology initiatives or projects related to electronic health records.

   (iii) Additional modeling of compensation strategy in the event such additional modeling is needed after completion of a Coker review pursuant to this Agreement regarding the sustainability of the current compensation plan.

   (iv) Required fair market value or opinion letters regarding compensation of physicians and other officers or employees.

   (v) Additional Client service line analysis or services unrelated to the Business as determined by Coker in its sole discretion.

   (vi) Additional medical staff development activities that are not related to the Business as determined by Coker in its sole discretion.

   (vii) Advisory services related to practice group acquisitions or mergers.

   (viii) Advisory services related to practice start-up services including, without limitation, expansion of Client developed pro form analysis.

   (ix) Functions and roles not normally associated with the POSITION's role in the Business as such role is commonly understood in the hospital industry.

In the event Client requests any of the Excluded Services, the parties will negotiate in good faith and execute a separate engagement letter outlining the services Coker will provide to Client and the fees that will be charged for such services. It is further agreed that this Agreement intends for Coker to provide some advisory services related to practice group acquisitions, mergers, and start-up services plus compensation analyses. However, the intent is that this should be limited to day-to-day, ongoing matters and not major initiatives akin to a separate project basis (which is the intent of the Excluded Services outlined above). In general, these will be defined as projects requiring significant off-site time by Coker corporate personnel or additional on-site time.

4. Duties of Client.

   (a) During the Term, Client shall remain validly formed and stay in good standing under the laws of the state of its formation and shall be qualified to do business in all other jurisdictions where such qualification is required.

   (b) No less frequently than at the end of each quarter during the calendar year, Client shall meet with a senior member of the Coker management team as designated by Coker for the purposes of discussing and remedying any operational issues that have arisen from the performance of the general management consulting services and POSITION services pursuant to the terms and conditions of this Agreement. Coker and Client further agree that there shall be a monthly meeting between Client, the POSITION and if, deemed necessary by Coker, in its sole discretion, a senior Coker management team member (participating via phone or in person). At such meeting Coker will submit a written report summarizing Coker's progress on the engagement in the past month and any operation issues that have arisen in such time period along with actions that will or will not be taken to address such issues. The Client's failure to hold the four quarterly meetings in a calendar year pursuant to this Section 4(b) will be considered a material breach of this Agreement by Client.

   (c) During the term of this Agreement and for a one year period after the termination of this Agreement for any reason, Client or its Affiliates may hire the ACTING POSITION or the POSITION provided by Coker pursuant to this Agreement and such Client or its Affiliate agrees to pay Coker $_____ as a recruiting fee for the recruitment and placement of the ACTING POSITION or the POSITION, as the case may be, with Client or its Affiliates and such recruiting fee is due upon the effective date that such ACTING POSITION or POSI-

TION begins employment with Client or its Affiliate. This Section 4(c) shall expressly survive termination of this Agreement for any reason.

5. <u>Events of Default by Coker.</u> Any of the following events or conditions shall constitute an event of default by Coker, if so declared by Client, in writing, (an "Coker Event of Default"): (a) Coker's default in performing any material obligation, term or condition of this Agreement, which default remains uncured for a period of sixty (60) days after Coker's receipt of written notice thereof from Client alleging such default and the specific actions necessary to remedy same; <u>provided, however</u>, that if such default is a nonmonetary default and cannot be cured within said sixty (60) day period, then Coker's cure period shall be extended until such default is cured so long as Coker, at all times during said cure period, diligently pursues curing such default; (b) upon the filing by or against Coker of a petition under any federal or state bankruptcy act or any amendment thereto or under any other insolvency or bankruptcy law or law providing for the relief of debtors, including, without limitation, a petition for reorganization, arrangement or extension; (c) upon the voluntary or involuntary making of an assignment of a substantial portion of its assets by Coker for the benefit of creditors, or the appointment of a receiver or trustee for Coker or for any of Coker's assets, or the institution by or against Coker of any other type of insolvency proceeding (under any federal or state bankruptcy act or otherwise) or of any formal or informal proceeding for dissolution, liquidation, settlement of claims against or winding up of the affairs of Coker, or the making by Coker of a transfer of all or a material portion of Coker's assets or inventory not in the ordinary course of business.

6. <u>Client's Remedies</u>. Upon a Coker Event of Default Client shall be entitled to terminate this Agreement upon notice to Coker whereupon Client shall be relieved of its obligations hereunder except for provisions of this Agreement that survive termination and to pursue such other rights and remedies as may be available at law or in equity, provided however, that Client must pay all fees Coker has earned pursuant to this Agreement through the termination date of this Agreement and Coker shall be entitled to any fees it earns or earned pursuant to Section 4(c).

7. <u>Events of Default by Client</u>. An event of default by Client (an "Client Event of Default") shall exist if any of the following occurs: (a) any failure by Client to pay Coker any amounts owed to Coker hereunder

when due and such monetary default remains uncured for a period of thirty (30) days after Client's receipt of written notice thereof from Coker describing the monetary default and the specific actions necessary to remedy such default ("Monetary Default"); (b) any other material breach of this Agreement by Client that is not a Monetary Default which default remains uncured for a period of sixty (60) days after Client's receipt of written notice thereof from Coker alleging such default and the specific actions necessary to remedy same; (c) upon the filing by or against Client of a petition under any federal or state bankruptcy act or any amendment thereto or under any other insolvency or bankruptcy law or law providing for the relief of debtors, including, without limitation, a petition for reorganization, arrangement or extension; or (d) upon the voluntary or involuntary making of an assignment of a substantial portion of its assets by Client for the benefit of creditors, or the appointment of a receiver or trustee for Client or for any of Client's assets, or the institution by or against Client of any other type of insolvency proceeding (under any federal or state bankruptcy act or otherwise) or of any formal or informal proceeding for dissolution, liquidation, settlement of claims against or winding up of the affairs of Client, or the making by Client of a transfer of all or a material portion of Client's assets or inventory not in the ordinary course of business.

8. Coker's Remedies. Upon the occurrence of a Client Event of Default, Coker, shall have the right to terminate this Agreement immediately by sending the Client notice of such termination, whereupon Coker shall be relieved from its obligations under this Agreement except for provisions of this Agreement that survive termination and to pursue such other rights and remedies as may be available to it at law or in equity, including, without limitation, receiving payment of the applicable termination fee in Section 2(h) as if Client terminated this Agreement pursuant to Section 1(c).

9. No Assignment. Neither party hereto shall have any right to assign, pledge, mortgage, transfer or otherwise dispose of, either in whole or in part, any of its rights, duties or obligations under this Agreement without having obtained the prior written consent of the other party hereto, and any attempt to do so without having obtained said prior written consent shall be null and void and of no force or effect whatsoever upon the other party.

10. Limitation on Liability of Coker. Client, its shareholders, officers, directors, employees, representatives, agents, predecessors, Affiliates,

successors and assigns ("Client Parties") hereby release and forever discharge Coker and its members, directors, manager, officers, employees, the ACTING POSITION, the POSITION representatives agents, predecessors, Affiliates, successors and assigns from any and all liability, claims, actions, causes of action, suits, demands, whether in law or in equity, whether known or unknown, for damages of every kind, character or description, expenses, or any costs whatsoever arising under any theory of liability against Client Parties that results from any action taken or for refraining from the taking of any action in good faith by the Coker Parties pursuant to this Agreement, or for good faith errors in judgment by the Coker Parties; *provided, however*, that this provision shall not protect Coker from any claim against Client that arises as a result of Coker's gross negligence or intentional misconduct in the performance of its duties and obligations pursuant to this Agreement. The Coker Parties are entitled to rely in good faith on any document of any kind prima facie properly executed and submitted by Client to Coker respecting any matters arising hereunder.

11. <u>Entire Agreement</u>. This Agreement contains the entire agreement between the parties pertaining to the subject matter hereof and supersedes all prior oral or written agreements between the parties with respect to said subject matter. No agreements, representations or understandings not specifically contained herein shall be binding upon any of the parties hereto. The terms, covenants, conditions and other provisions of this Agreement may hereafter be changed, amended or modified only by an instrument in writing specifically purporting so to do and signed by the party against whom enforcement is sought.

12. <u>Notices</u>. All communications or notices required or permitted by this Agreement shall be in writing and shall be deemed to have been given (i) on the date of personal delivery to an officer of or personally to the other party, or (ii) when sent by telecopy or facsimile machine to the number shown below on the date of such confirmed facsimile or telecopy transmission provided a copy is also sent pursuant to overnight delivery with a nationallyrecognized commercial overnight delivery service as pursuant to (iii) of this Section or (iii) the day following deposit when properly deposited for overnight delivery with a nationallyrecognized commercial overnight delivery service, prepaid, or by deposit in the United States mail, certified or registered mail, postage prepaid, return receipt requested on the date that is two (2) days after the date set forth on the return receipt, and addressed as follows, unless and until either of such parties notifies the other in accordance with this

Section of a change of address or change of telecopy number:

To Coker:
    Coker Group Holdings, LLC
    Max Reiboldt, CPA
    President/CEO
    2400 Lakeview Parkway, Suite 400
    Alpharetta, Georgia 30009
    Facsimile: (678) 832 2016

with a copy to:

and if to Client:
    ABC Hospital
    Attention: President
    1000 Elm Street
    Anywhere, State 00000
    Facsimile: _____

with a copy to:
    _____
    Attention: _____
    _____
    _____
    Facsimile: _____

13. <u>Binding Effect; Amendment and Waiver</u>. This Agreement shall be binding upon and inure to the benefit of the parties and their respective successors and assigns. No amendment, supplement, modification, or waiver of this Agreement shall be binding unless executed in writing by the party to be bound thereby. No waiver of any of the provisions of this Agreement shall be deemed or shall constitute a waiver of any other provision of this Agreement, whether or not similar, unless otherwise expressly provided. No failure on the part of any party hereto to exercise and no delay in exercising any right, power or remedy hereunder shall operate as a waiver thereof, nor shall any single or partial exercise of any right, power or remedy hereunder preclude any other or further exercise thereof or the exercise of any other right, power or remedy.

14. Counterparts; Headings. This Agreement may be executed in several counterparts, each of which shall be deemed an original, but such counterparts shall together constitute but one and the same Agreement. This Agreement may be executed and delivered in counterpart signature pages executed and delivered via facsimile transmission, and any such counterpart executed and delivered via facsimile transmission shall be deemed an original for all intents and purposes.

15. Severability. If any provision, clause or part of this Agreement or the application thereof under certain circumstances is held invalid or unenforceable, the remainder of this Agreement, or the application of such provision, clause or part under other circumstances, shall not be affected thereby.

16. Governing Law. This Agreement shall be construed and interpreted according to the laws of the State of Georgia, without regard to the conflict of law principles thereof. The parties agree and consent to the jurisdiction of the Federal and State Courts of Fulton County, Georgia and waive jurisdiction and venue in any other court.

17. Saturdays, Sundays and Legal Holidays. If the time period by which any acts or payments required hereunder must be performed or paid expires on a Saturday, Sunday or legal holiday, then such time period shall be automatically extended to the close of business on the next regularly scheduled business day.

18. Time is of the Essence. Time is of the essence with respect to this Agreement.

19. Judicial Interpretation. Should any provision of this Agreement require judicial interpretation, the parties hereto agree that the court interpreting or construing the same shall not apply a presumption that the terms hereof shall be more strictly construed against one party by reason of the rule of construction that a document is to be construed more strictly against the party which itself or through its agent prepared the same, it being agreed that the agents of each party have participated in the preparation hereof.

20. Dispute Resolution/Mediation. The parties agree to work together in good faith to resolve all disputes and controversies under this Agreement for a period of thirty (30) days after either party notifies the other of the dispute or controversy along with a brief explanation of such dispute or controversy. In the event the parties are unable to resolve the dispute or controversy then all disputes and controversies of every

kind and nature between the parties to this Agreement arising out of or in connection with the existence, construction, validity, interpretation or meaning, performance, non- performance, enforcement, operation, breach, continuance, or termination of the Agreement shall first be submitted to mediation pursuant to the procedure set forth in this Section 20. The Client or Coker may demand such mediation immediately in writing after the parties are unable to amicably resolve their differences within thirty (30) day period. The parties agree that the mediator shall be appointed by the Atlanta office of the Judicial Arbitration and Mediation Services, Inc. (JAMS) and shall be held in JAMS Atlanta office. The mediation shall be concluded within thirty (30) days of the selection of the mediator. The parties shall equally bear the cost of the mediator but otherwise bear their own costs in connection with the mediation.

21. <u>Independent Contractor</u>. Coker shall be deemed to be an independent contractor in the performance of the services contemplated by this Agreement and shall not be considered or permitted to be an agent, servant, joint venturer or partner of Client. At no time shall Coker and Client be considered to be co-employers or joint employers.

22. <u>Attorney Fees</u>. In the event of a breach of this Agreement, the non-breaching party may recover its reasonable attorney fees actually incurred from the breaching party in addition to any other damages it is entitled to recover pursuant to this Agreement or Georgia and Federal law.

23. <u>Affiliates Definition</u>. For purposes of this Agreement, Affiliates shall mean any person, corporation, partnership, limited liability company, trust or other entity controlling, controlled by or under common control with the Client; or any officer, director, trustee, partner, member, manager or holder of ten percent (10 percent) or more of the outstanding voting securities of any corporation, partnership, limited liability company, trust or other entity controlling, controlled by or under common control with the Client.

[SIGNATURES ON THE FOLLOWING PAGE]

IN WITNESS WHEREOF, the undersigned parties, acting by and through their respective duly authorized officers, have executed this Agreement, and caused their corporate seals to be affixed hereto, all as of the day and year first above written.

COKER GROUP HOLDINGS, LLC

, a Georgia Limited Liability Company

By: _____
              Max Reiboldt, CPA
              President/CEO

[CORPORATE SEAL]

CLIENT

ABC HOSPITAL, a STATE Non-Profit Corporation

By: _____
Name: _____
Title:_____

[CORPORATE SEAL]

SECTION 2

CHAPTER 1

Overview of Stage I Alignment

As noted in Section I of this book, the healthcare industry is experiencing rapid and radical changes, and both private practices and health systems are being forced to adapt to survive. The main impetus for the change stems from the introduction of population health management and the shift to the provision of value-based services and patient-centered healthcare. Previously, we outlined the changes to the compensation and reimbursement models relevant to this industry shift; however, the other more encompassing shift is in the structure of the organizations themselves. In an article in *Modern Healthcare*, it was reported that "hospital ownership of physician practices has increased by 86% in the last three years" and "physicians employed by hospitals increased by 50%" in the same period. Alternatively, 62% of physicians in the United States are not employed by a hospital or system.[1] While that may seem like a large percentage of independent providers, that statistic does not take into account the other methods of alignment for physicians.

This momentum is driving providers and hospitals to align and to integrate in the most mutually beneficial fashion available, thereby creating a spectrum of alignment and integration options. Figure 2.1.1, Stage 1 Alignment Models, illustrates these various models, ranging from limited to full integration. In this chapter, we will detail a few key structures and compare their benefits and drawbacks.

It is important to note that we consider all of these structures to be Stage I of alignment or financial integration, with Stage II being clinical integration. We will delve into Stage II in later chapters; however, it is important to see these structures as building toward further integra-

Limited Integration	Moderate Integration	Full Integration
Managed Care Networks (Independent Practice Associations, Physician Hospital Organizations): Loose alliances for contracting purposes	Service Line Management: Management of all specialty services within the hospital	ACO/CIN/QC: Participation in an organization focused on improving quality/cost of care for governmental or non-governmental payers; may be driven by practices or hospital/groups
Recruitment/Incubation: Economic assistance for new physicians	MSO/ISO: Ties hospitals to physician's business	Employment "Lite": Professional services agreements (PSAs) and other similar models (such as the practice management arrangement) through which hospital engages physicians as contractors
Group (Legal-Only) Merger: Unites parties under common legal entity without an operational merger	Clinical Co-Management: Physicians become actively engaged in clinical operations and oversight of applicable service line at the hospital	
Call Coverage Stipends: Pay for unassigned ED call	Equity Group Assimilation: Ties entities via legal agreement; joint practice ownership	Employment*: Strongest alignment; minimizes economic risk for physicians;
Medical Directorships: Specific clinical oversight duties	Joint Ventures: Unites parties under common enterprise; difficult to structure; legal hurdles	Group (Legal and Operational) Merger: Unites parties under common legal entity with full integration of operations

■ Typically Physician-to-Physician   ■ Typically Physician-to-Hospital   ■ Either Physician-Physician or Physician-Hospital

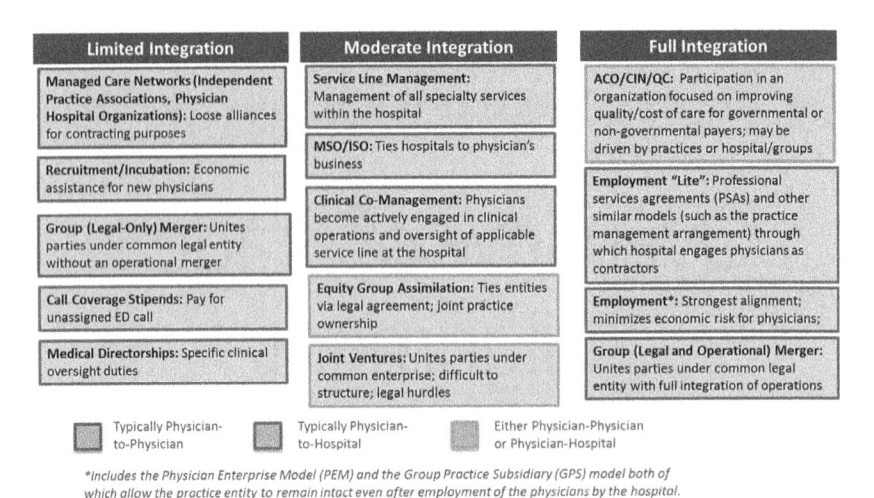

*Includes the Physician Enterprise Model (PEM) and the Group Practice Subsidiary (GPS) model both of which allow the practice entity to remain intact even after employment of the physicians by the hospital.

FIGURE 2.1.1 Stage 1 Alignment Models

tion. Through alignment, organizations are aligned via common goals and objectives, and it tends to be a more structural than functional relationship. Essentially, Stage I is simply how two entities become tied together by legal and economic connections.

Stage II is the second step of alignment for an overall Accountable Care Era strategy. Through clinical integration, the entities become a fully merged clinical and business model, thereby being more functional than structural entities. Moreover, Stage II represents the organizations becoming tied together by clinical and cultural connections and presents the opportunity to capitalize fully on the nuances of value-based care.

Again, we will focus on Stage II in later chapters, outlining the structures that can be included in this second step, but first, we will focus on Stage I of alignment.

PHYSICIAN-TO-HOSPITAL ALIGNMENT MODELS— STAGE I (FINANCIAL INTEGRATION)

Both hospitals and physicians can benefit from alignment and integration; however, the two parties may have different motives. Hospitals are seeking to bridge gaps in care (especially of particular concern in rural areas) and sustain or grow their current market status. Physicians are looking for ways to mitigate reduced reimbursement, increased management requirements, and rising overhead costs; however, physi-

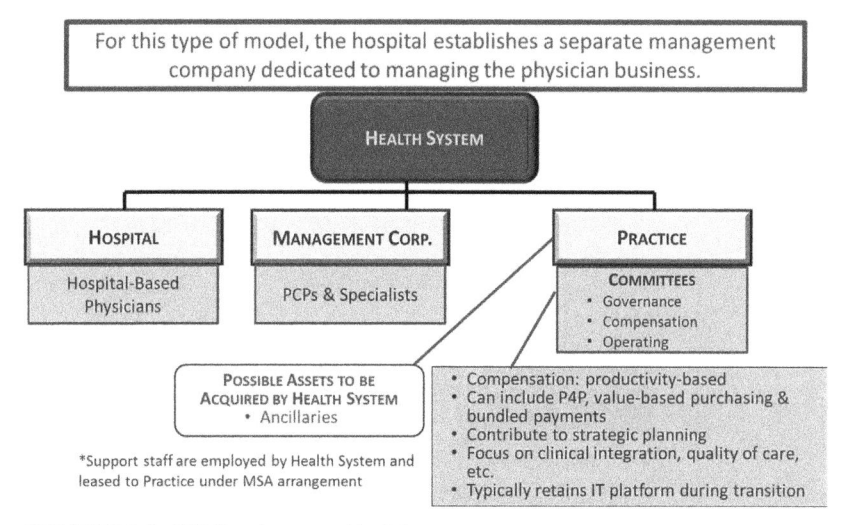

```
┌─────────────────────────────────────────────────────────────┐
│ For this type of model, the hospital establishes a separate │
│ management company dedicated to managing the physician      │
│ business.                                                   │
└─────────────────────────────────────────────────────────────┘
                         HEALTH SYSTEM
          ┌──────────────────┼──────────────────┐
       HOSPITAL        MANAGEMENT CORP.      PRACTICE
    Hospital-Based     PCPs & Specialists    COMMITTEES
     Physicians                              • Governance
                                             • Compensation
                                             • Operating

    POSSIBLE ASSETS TO BE          • Compensation: productivity-based
    ACQUIRED BY HEALTH SYSTEM      • Can include P4P, value-based purchasing &
      • Ancillaries                  bundled payments
                                   • Contribute to strategic planning
*Support staff are employed by     • Focus on clinical integration, quality of care,
 Health System and leased to         etc.
 Practice under MSA arrangement    • Typically retains IT platform during transition
```

FIGURE 2.1.2 GPS Employment Model

cians are extremely focused on retaining control of their businesses. Therefore, to satisfy both parties, all alignment models—not just employment—should be considered.

Employment

Employment is still the most encompassing form of integration, offering a breadth of benefits to both physicians and hospitals. The common employment structure involves an employment agreement between a physician and hospital, benefits provided to the physician and paid for by the hospital, as well as the standard employee regulations, and less flexibility and autonomy, but with the potential for more job security. There are, however, several alternative forms of employment: the group practice subsidiary (GPS), the group without walls (GWW), and the joint management (Dyad) models.

1. **GPS:** The hospital employs all physicians from a private practice en masse; the practice functions as a cohesive, separate subsidiary entity with a high level of independence and autonomy, even within a broader employed physician network model. The GPS model is illustrated in Figure 2.1.2.
2. **GWW:** The hospital establishes a separate management company dedicated to managing the physician businesses; physicians retain separate offices and finances. Often a central business office is estab-

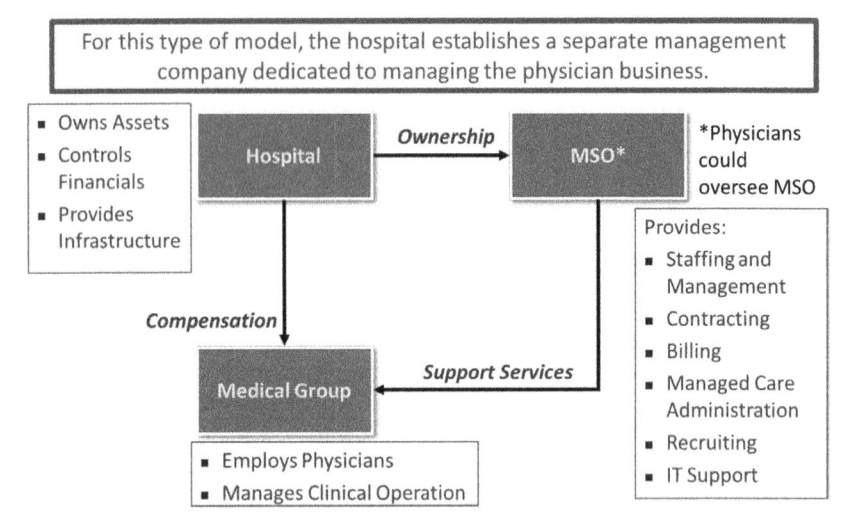

FIGURE 2.1.3. GWW Employment Model

Diagram description:
- Header: For this type of model, the hospital establishes a separate management company dedicated to managing the physician business.
- Hospital: Owns Assets, Controls Financials, Provides Infrastructure
- Hospital → (Ownership) → MSO* (*Physicians could oversee MSO)
- Hospital → (Compensation) → Medical Group
- MSO → (Support Services) → Medical Group
- MSO Provides: Staffing and Management, Contracting, Billing, Managed Care Administration, Recruiting, IT Support
- Medical Group: Employs Physicians, Manages Clinical Operation

lished to house administrative services and some or all ancillary services. The GWW model illustrated in Figure 2.1.3.

3. **Dyad:** Common in larger employed networks, this model involves dedicated administrative oversight, but frequently segregated physicians, by service area. In the most common variant of the model, physicians are organized by specialty, with a physician leader paired with an administrative leader to ensure the group has sufficient bandwidth and focus on both clinical and business goals. Figure 2.1.4 illustrates the Dyad model.

The primary benefit to pursuing a full employment relationship for physicians is the overhead support and stability that a hospital can provide. Many physicians feel as though running the business side of their practices is not something they excel in or even enjoy; thus, utilizing a hospital allows them to focus on their areas of expertise. However, with stability comes some level of oversight that private practice physicians may not be accustomed to having. Depending on the hospital and contract, varying degrees of clinical oversight will remain, but the physicians likely will no longer be determining other decisions such as personnel staffing, scheduling, equipment and supply vendors, etc. Thus, while employment may be a viable option for some practices, it is important to note that other (non-employment) options are available that allow more flexibility and control.

Chapter 1—Overview of Stage I Alignment   **121**

> The network model typically has dedicated oversight but frequently segregates physicians by service focus.

```
Hospital CEO
    ↓
Physician Network CEO  →  Network Planning + Clinical Coordination
```

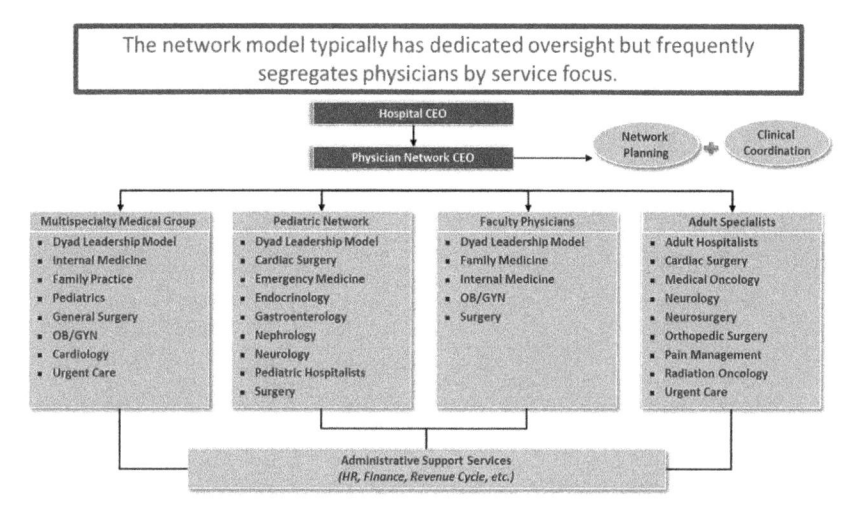

Multispecialty Medical Group	Pediatric Network	Faculty Physicians	Adult Specialists
• Dyad Leadership Model	• Dyad Leadership Model	• Dyad Leadership Model	• Adult Hospitalists
• Internal Medicine	• Cardiac Surgery	• Family Medicine	• Cardiac Surgery
• Family Practice	• Emergency Medicine	• Internal Medicine	• Medical Oncology
• Pediatrics	• Endocrinology	• OB/GYN	• Neurology
• General Surgery	• Gastroenterology	• Surgery	• Neurosurgery
• OB/GYN	• Nephrology		• Orthopedic Surgery
• Cardiology	• Neurology		• Pain Management
• Urgent Care	• Pediatric Hospitalists		• Radiation Oncology
	• Surgery		• Urgent Care

Administrative Support Services
(HR, Finance, Revenue Cycle, etc.)

FIGURE 2.1.4 Dyad Employment Model

Clinical Co-Management Agreement

Clinical Co-management Agreements (CCMAs) offer an alternative to employment or a Professional Services Agreement (described below), while still serving as a form of moderate alignment between two parties (likely a hospital and private practice). More specifically, CCMAs are a way for hospital service lines to utilize a private practice for clinical and operational oversight, while providing a stable and rewarding relationship for the practice's providers.

These agreements are structured via a contractual relationship between the hospital and management entity to reward physicians for their efforts in developing, managing, and improving the quality and efficiency of the hospital's service line. The scope of such agreements may cover multi-site, inpatient, outpatient, and/or ancillary services. In this type of arrangement, provider compensation is based on a hybrid of performance-based incentives, such as achievement of specific quality objectives and potentially shared cost savings. Additionally, a CCMA can be structured either as a standalone arrangement or included in conjunction with a full alignment transaction in the form of a "wraparound" agreement. A general CCMA structure is shown in Figure 2.1.5.

Like other alignment structures, a CCMA can be structured in several different forms, as noted below.

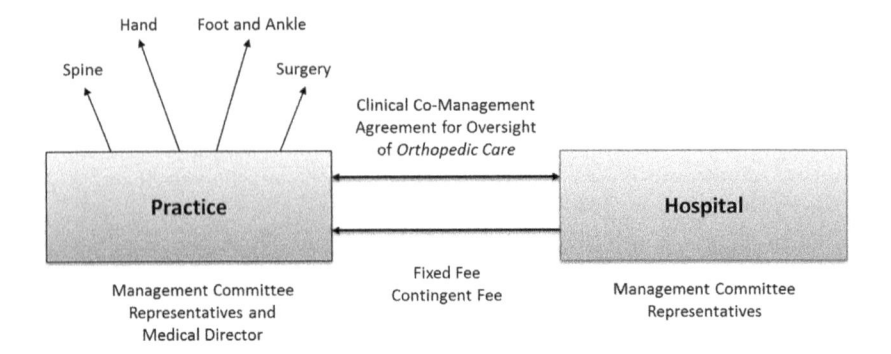

```
    Hand    Foot and Ankle
Spine         Surgery
                        Clinical Co-Management
                        Agreement for Oversight
                          of *Orthopedic Care*

    [Practice]  ←——————→  [Hospital]

                         Fixed Fee
Management Committee    Contingent Fee    Management Committee
Representatives and                       Representatives
Medical Director
```

Each service line/specialty can have its own CCMA, which can be included as a singular alignment strategy or as a "wraparound" (i.e., add-on) to another, major alignment strategy

FIGURE 2.1.5 CCMA Example

1. ***Traditional CCMA:*** This model consists of a management agreement between an existing physician professional corporation and a hospital or its service line.
2. ***Newly Created Entity CCMA:*** This model is structured by the development of a newly created management entity by a physician-owned group, which then enters into a management agreement with a hospital or its service line.
3. ***Joint Venture CCMA:*** A Joint Venture CCMA is made up of a physician-owned group and a hospital that merge to create a Joint Venture management entity. This Joint Venture management entity then enters into a management agreement with a hospital or its service line.
4. ***Joint Oversight CCMA:*** A Joint Oversight CCMA structure comprises two or more physician groups that together create a Joint Oversight Committee with which a hospital coordinates services.

A CCMA is a viable strategy for those entities that are interested in pursuing a more integrated relationship with a hospital but are not necessarily ready to align fully. Additionally, it serves as an excellent vehicle for physicians to become more involved in the clinical and administrative oversight of their service line. CCMAs can be somewhat difficult to structure, as the hospital will have to fund additional compensation for these activities or utilize shared savings as a source of funding.

CCMAs continue to gain traction as a repose to the Accountable Care Era and as organizations face increased pressure to improve quality and reduce costs, thereby being compelled to utilize their private practice counterparts for physician input and influence.

Employment Lite

"Employment lite" is a term often used to describe a physician-hospital alignment model that falls just short of full employment. As opposed to a "W-2" relationship, it is commonly a "1099" contracted position, formalized by a Professional Services Agreement (PSA). Under the employment lite arrangement, a hospital contractually engages a physician or practice to provide certain services. While these arrangements are similar to full employment in the day-to-day operations of the business, the legal and financial structures tend to allow more flexibility for the practice/physicians. The agreement may include solely clinical (professional) services or may also encompass "wraparounds" (such as administrative duties, unassigned ED call coverage, etc.). Many clinical-only PSAs are paid based on wRVU productivity with a separate payment to cover overhead expenses. However, wraparounds can take other forms of payment (hourly stipend, daily stipend, etc.). Below are descriptions of four conventional PSA structures, illustrated in Figures 2.1.6–2.1.9.

1. ***Traditional PSA:*** The hospital contracts with physicians for professional services; the hospital employs staff and "owns" the administrative structure (see Figure 2.1.6).
2. ***Global Payment PSA:*** The hospital contracts with practice for services in exchange for a global payment rate, which includes all physician compensation and benefits as well as all practice overhead expenses; the practice retains all management responsibilities (see Figure 2.1.7).
3. ***Practice Management Arrangement (PMA):*** The hospital employs physicians; the practice entity is preserved and contracts with the hospital for management services; administrative management staff are not employed by the hospital, as the practice provides these services via a management contract and receives a corresponding fee (see Figure 2.1.8).
4. ***Hybrid Model:*** Overall, the PSA model can take many forms, as various scenarios involving "mixing/matching" of services (both professional and administrative) exist (see Figure 2.1.9).

Traditional PSA Model

Hospital/Health System:
- Assumes responsibility for Practice's management and operations (includes lease/depreciation expense and other operating expenses) → Deducted from professional service revenue to be paid to Practice
- Pays the Practice's real estate lease → Lease expense deducted from professional service revenue to be paid to Practice
- Purchases or leases ancillary services; bills HOPD rates → Fixed payment (upfront or annually) to the Practice, set in advance
- Employs Practice staff (both ancillary and non-ancillary staff) → Fully loaded expense deducted from professional service revenue to be paid to Practice
- Contracts directly with payers for professional and technical fees

Independent Contractor

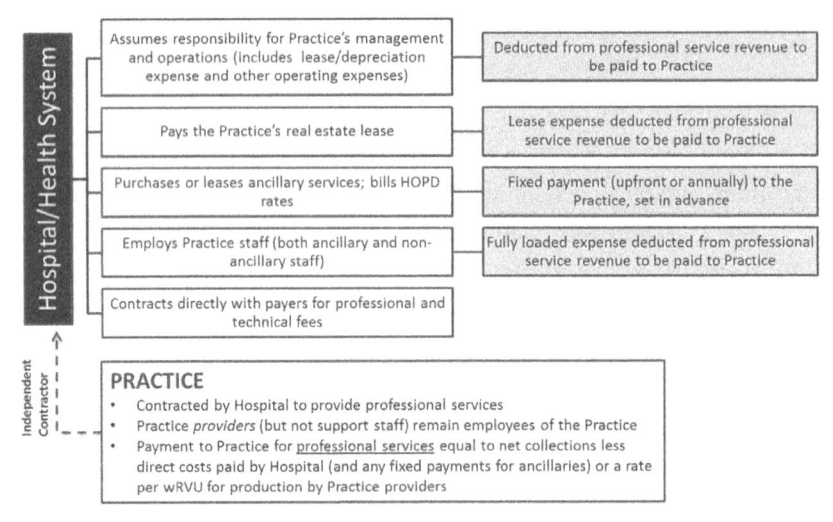

PRACTICE
- Contracted by Hospital to provide professional services
- Practice *providers* (but not support staff) remain employees of the Practice
- Payment to Practice for <u>professional services</u> equal to net collections less direct costs paid by Hospital (and any fixed payments for ancillaries) or a rate per wRVU for production by Practice providers

FIGURE 2.1.6 Traditional PSA Model

Global Payment PSA Model

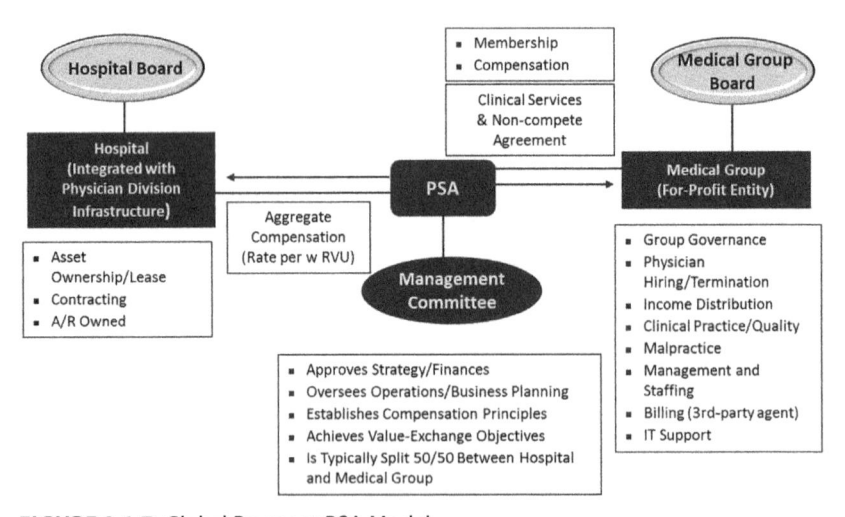

Hospital Board — **Hospital (Integrated with Physician Division Infrastructure)**
- Asset Ownership/Lease
- Contracting
- A/R Owned

PSA (between Hospital and Medical Group)
- Membership
- Compensation
- Clinical Services & Non-compete Agreement
- Aggregate Compensation (Rate per wRVU)

Management Committee
- Approves Strategy/Finances
- Oversees Operations/Business Planning
- Establishes Compensation Principles
- Achieves Value-Exchange Objectives
- Is Typically Split 50/50 Between Hospital and Medical Group

Medical Group Board — **Medical Group (For-Profit Entity)**
- Group Governance
- Physician Hiring/Termination
- Income Distribution
- Clinical Practice/Quality
- Malpractice
- Management and Staffing
- Billing (3rd-party agent)
- IT Support

FIGURE 2.1.7 Global Payment PSA Model

PSA models offer significant advantages. Hospitals can partner in a meaningful way with physicians without the perceived challenges that often accompany employment. These structures provide ample flexibility, but they also can prove to be a viable segue into full employment if desired by the parties. Both the hospital and practice can increase volume and revenue while controlling costs.

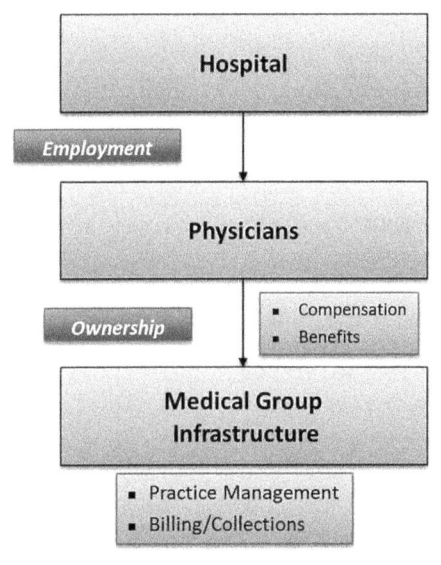

FIGURE 2.1.8 Practice Management Arrangement PSA Model

In general, a PSA strategy poses fewer disadvantages than advantages, but some are still important to note. Inherently, these structures are less stable than employment and could be more easily terminated by either party. Moreover, these arrangements require high levels of commitment, therefore inhibiting the overall ability for the practice to partner or engage with other facilities. Occasionally, issues with management may arise as administrative and professional services may be handled separately. Information technology integration/transition cannot only prove to be both costly and add gaps in the timeline, but can also cause one or both organizations to incur sunk costs during the conversion. Hospitals often perceive a lack of control, but in reality, if properly structured, this is no different than employment.

Joint Equity Ventures

Joint Equity Ventures (JEVs) represent another innovative strategy to responding to the financial pressures of the Accountable Care Era and are illustrated in Figure 2.1.10. JEVs can take various structures, including physician-to-physician or physician-to-third-party investor models. Most commonly, these are project-driven entities for the development of new capital struc-

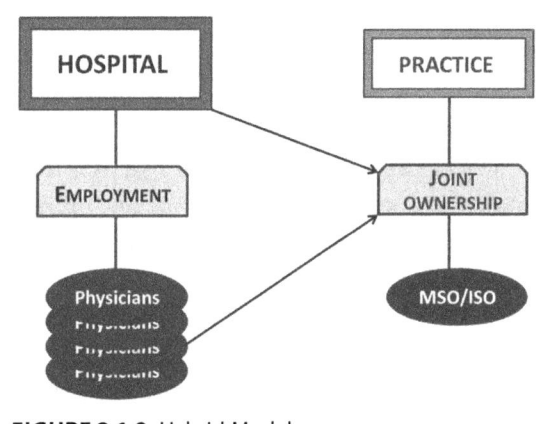

FIGURE 2.1.9 Hybrid Model

```
┌─────────────┐      ┌─────────────┐
│  Hospital   │  ✚   │  Practice   │
└─────────────┘      └─────────────┘
```

Legally permissible if one of the following is met:
1. Physicians contribute financial capital
2. Physicians provided business expertise
3. Physicians assume business risk

Possible Structures*
- Specialty Hospitals
- Management Services Arrangement
- Under Arrangement Arrangements
- Freestanding Centers (i.e. MOB or ASC)
- Pay for Performance
- Block Leases
- Medical Directorships

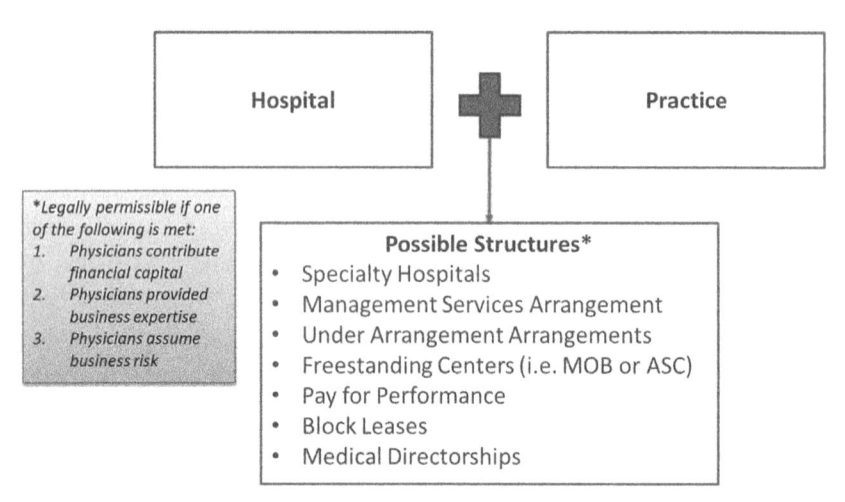

FIGURE 2.1.10 Joint Equity Venture

tures, such as an ambulatory surgery center. However, JEVs also can be for management services arrangements, leases, medical directorships, and other structures. In most scenarios, the two entities share oversight of the project; however, if one entity is more financially invested, it might hold the overall authority on decisions. Either way, JEVs can be helpful in combining the market presence, financial capital, and stability of a hospital with the clinical oversight and reputation of a private practice or physician.

For physicians, a JEV can provide a separate source of income in the face of decreasing reimbursement and more focus on value-based care. This factor can be an attractive recruiting principal for hospitals if they have a potential JEV to offer employees or physician partners. Additionally, it can provide an avenue for both the physicians and the hospital to consider the expansion of their current service offerings or an addition of ancillary services.

The primary consideration for JEVs is the applicable laws and regulations to consider, including but not limited to Stark, Anti-Kickback Statutes, and state laws. For a JEV to be legally permissible, one of the following items should be met (1) physicians contribute financial capital to the JEV, (2) physicians provide business expertise for the hospital, or (3) physicians have an inherent business risk associated with the structure. When considering a JEV, substantial thought should be given to all associated laws and regulations.

PHYSICIAN-TO-PHYSICIAN ALIGNMENT MODELS—
STAGE I (FINANCIAL INTEGRATION)

While we have previously discussed the benefits and stability afforded to physicians and private practices that decide to pursue alignment with a hospital, it is also important to highlight the potential for physician practices to align with their peers to counter decreasing compensation and reimbursement. One of the many benefits of the Accountable Care Era is the increasingly popular structures that have become possible for physician collaboratives as a response to these industry changes. Moreover, none of these are "one-size-fits-all" arrangements and may be altered or combined to best suit the practice.

Recruitment

Recruitment is a relatively straightforward concept for increasing the market share and presence of a private practice. With increased size comes increased stability and the ability to negotiate with payers and hospitals. Moreover, this alignment strategy is accessible to all practices, regardless of size, as it requires minimal up-front capital. Additionally, recruitment can be as small as growing by a single provider, or it could become a comprehensive strategy wherein the practice grows to a large multispecialty clinic with extensive ancillary service offerings.

1. ***Single-Specialty Practice:*** Single-specialty practices can include either a handful of providers in the same office or a large group of providers spanning multiple facilities. It can begin with a gradual increase of providers within an existing practice or a merger with one or more other practices of the same specialty (described in more detail below). Likely, the group would share practice profits as well as some of the costs related to facilities, equipment, and employees.
2. ***Multispecialty Practice:*** Again, a multispecialty practice could be developed through organic growth of additional providers or a merger of multispecialty practices. Ideally, the multispecialty practice would begin with a strong primary care base wherein these primary care physicians could provide a continual stream of referrals to specialists within the practice.

Recruitment is an attractive alignment strategy as it requires little start-up capital and does not exclude the practice from participating in

1. Legal Merger
- The development of a new legal entity either through the creation of a "NewCo," or Practice A "merging" into Practice B (or vice versa)
- All groups under one TIN but operating much the same as today, with some exceptions
- A "pod" mentality often exists under a legally merged structure

2. Operational Merger
- Operations, economics, governance are consolidated within NewCo
- Once established, standardization across most functional areas (clinical and business) within NewCo occurs
- A full operational merger can be effectuated by an initial legal merger phase followed by operational merger that occurs over time

To confuse things further, hybrid structures are also possible!

FIGURE 2.1.11 Mergers

other alignment strategies at the same time or in the future. However, practices should ensure that physicians are a good clinical fit, as they likely will become partners in the practice, thereby becoming equally involved in all clinical and administrative considerations.

Mergers

As noted above, both single-specialty and multispecialty practices can be formed through mergers. Mergers typically fit into two major categories: legal-only mergers and operational mergers; however, hybrid structures are also possible. These structures are outlined in Figure 2.1.11.

1. *Legal-Only Merger:* The legal-only merger is defined through the development of a new legal entity, through either the creation of a new practice (NewCo) or a merger of one practice into another. All groups would bill under a single tax ID number; however, little else would change regarding day-to-day operations. A "pod" mentality often exists under a legally merged structure where practices are operating in their sole best intentions, with little regard for their other practices.
2. *Operational Merger:* Under an operational merger, operations, economics, and governance are all consolidated within NewCo.

Once established, standardization across most functional areas, both clinical and business, within NewCo occurs. This transaction can happen immediately, or an initial legal merger phase can be followed by an operational merger that occurs over time.

Some considerations should be made in both scenarios before entering into a merger agreement. Some major global issues include structural, operational, relational, governance, financial, physical facility, or clinical considerations. It is crucial to vet all of these issues to the greatest extent possible before making a decision, as this structure is relatively complicated to unwind.

If all of these issues are fully vetted, and the practices agree to further their relationship via a merger, this arrangement can provide a relatively quick solution for growing a practice. A merger can help practices respond to value-based care through expanded resources, gain better bargaining power with both hospitals and payers, and establish a more dominant market presence.

In facilitating mergers for our clients, we typically follow the steps listed below and illustrated in Figure 2.1.12.

1. Identify potential partners and ascertain the goals of each organization;
2. Determine merger readiness and isolate key issues (both individually and collectively);

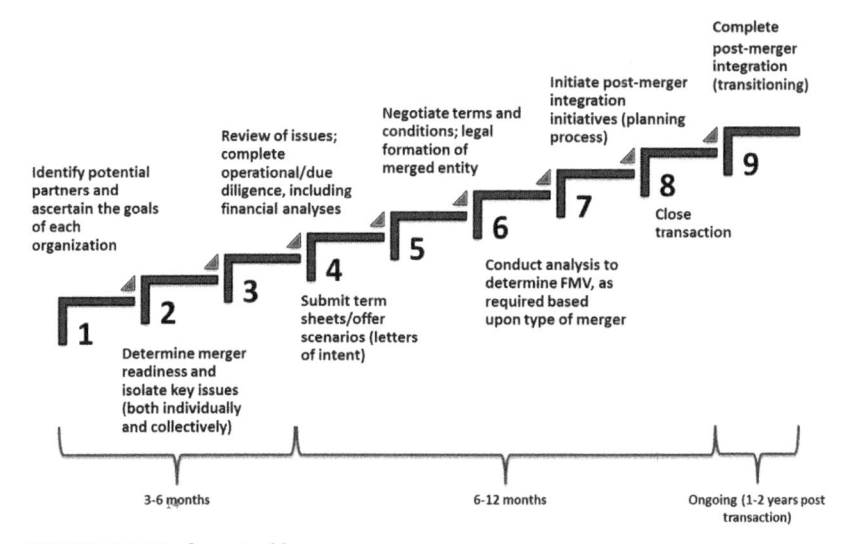

FIGURE 2.1.12 Steps to Merger

3. Review issues and complete operational/due diligence, including financial analyses;
4. Submit term sheets/offer scenarios (i.e., letters of intent);
5. Negotiate terms and conditions and legally form merged entity;
6. Conduct analysis to determine FMV, as required based on type of merger;
7. Initiate post-merger integration initiatives (planning process);
8. Close transaction; and
9. Complete post-merger integration (transitioning).

Private Practice Collaboratives

This final alignment strategy is incredibly innovative and is an excellent building block to further integrations (i.e., Stage II – Clinical Integration). These physician collaboratives can be entirely independent of hospital interaction through an independent practice association (IPA) or can combine a physician collaborative with a hospital to create a physician-hospital organization (PHO).

Under these structures, physicians seek to use the current challenges in the healthcare industry as an opportunity to improve patient care and the practice environment for themselves. For these entities to be successful, they must establish some core tenets of integration. They should seek to design highly reliable, cost-efficient, evidence-based, and patient-centric processes of care. The processes and protocols should be monitored via the measurement of outcomes to determine the true value of care being delivered. Additionally, data metrics should be used to drive continuous value improvement and to create a true learning organization. Further, all of these initiatives should be governed by a system of accountability that holds all providers to the physician-determined standards of care, cost and quality goals, and overall clinical ideals.

The key with physician collaboratives is to respond to market changes by collaborating with local providers as partners to lay the foundation for integrated care. It can provide an opportunity to maximize revenue and take advantage of economies of scale. Moreover, it can boost the physician base to ensure adequate continuums of care and primary care development. However, as with all alignment structures, there are key legal and regulatory considerations to take into account, specifically pertaining to compensation and payer contracting negotiations. Thus, all parties should understand and fully vet the motivations for participating in such a collaborative before entering into such an arrangement.

We will discuss the concept of Stage II alignment models in more detail in the following chapter. Nevertheless, it is important to understand that a form of physician collaboratives can be a clinically integrated organization such as a clinically integrated network (CIN), accountable care organization (ACO), quality collaborative (QC), or patient-centered medical home (PCMH). Clinically integrated organizations, or Stage II alignment models, are structures that are legally and clinically integrated to respond to create a continuum of care that serves to increase the quality of care for patients while reducing the burden of costs placed on physicians, payers, and even patients. Each of the physician collaboratives outlined above can be built upon to create a successful clinically integrated organization; however, they may lead to a variation of the structure. Again, more details will be presented in later chapters.

PHYSICIAN COMPENSATION FOR STAGE I ALIGNMENT STRUCTURES

As we noted in previous chapters, the shift from volume- to value-based reimbursement has led to a mirrored shift in how physicians are compensated. While this change will affect employed physicians a good deal, essentially all of the alignment structures outlined above include some form of compensation in the contract, whether physicians seek to align with a private practice or a hospital. The industry likely will continue to see increased focus on fee-for-value measures going forward.

For example, for CCMAs, the hospital partner likely will tie certain incentives to the formation of value-based care initiatives and PSAs will incorporate aspects of quality and cost metrics in the compensation or reimbursement structure. JEVs will seek to establish themselves as a low-cost provider, utilizing physician input to control such measures. For private practice collaborations, there likely will be high involvement in value-based reimbursement plans, leading to the potential for shared savings to be allocated among the physicians. Moreover, as the alignment structures move into Stage II, there will be even more pressure to create organizations that are focused on the *value* of care rather than just the volume, thereby leading to altered incentives for physicians.

CONCLUSION

Many of the contracts in place today, with other private practices or with hospital partners, are nearing the end of their initial term. Thus, many organizations are facing the question of how best to adapt their current structure to respond to the Accountable Care Era. Hence, the industry is seeing an increase in practices and hospitals interested in pursuing Stage II alignment. Still, other practices are moving toward the second generation of their original contract, with more focus on value-based incentives and further integration with their partners.

For those organizations interested in pursuing the clinical integration function of alignment (i.e., Stage II), some important considerations should be discussed. First, the organization should understand its individual market, as certain locations are moving more slowly toward these forms of value-based care. Payer mix is another significant point of consideration, as commercial payers are moving more quickly toward these value-based reimbursement models; however, a strong private payer mix will create more leverage in negotiations. Finally, the individual entity and its providers should be considered. The key to any successful clinical integration strategy lies with the physicians, as they will need to both support the initiative and to drive it. These matters will be discussed in more detail in the following chapters; however, it is important to note that clinical integration is not always the answer.

Either way, the current healthcare market has compelled physicians and hospitals to search for strategic alignment solutions. While many are still moving toward full employment, a high percentage of physicians and healthcare systems are seeking other options that suit their particular situation more effectively, including pursuing strategies for clinical integration. The ultimate goal is for hospitals and physicians to incorporate both traditional and contemporary alignment aspects to meet the needs of the shifting healthcare landscape.

REFERENCE

1. Castellucci M. Hospital ownership of medical practices grows by 86% in three years. *Modern Healthcare.* September 2016. http://www.modernhealthcare.com/article/20160907/NEWS/160909936. Accessed October 21, 2016.

SECTION II

CHAPTER 2

Market/Industry Dynamics Promoting Stage II Alignment

As the ACA and MACRA facilitate the transition of the healthcare industry from fee-for-service payments to value-based payments, new alignment models must strive to provide value (i.e., improve quality and reduce costs) in the provision of healthcare services. Many quality issues that alignment models seek to address are access to healthcare, increased coordination of healthcare services, patient-centric care, and high-risk care that jeopardizes patient safety. Also, these alignment structures need to accommodate efforts by providers to scrutinize costs systematically and eliminate those that increase expenses but do not add to quality outcomes.

Quality Improvements in the Value-Based Reimbursement Era

Improving the population's access to healthcare services can have one of the biggest impacts on the quality the alignment model provides to its community. Access to healthcare services is "the timely use of personal health services to achieve the best health outcomes."[1] Three of the biggest reasons for the lack of access to quality healthcare services is the lack of available services in a person's geographic area, the high cost of these services, and an individual's lack of insurance coverage.

Many alignment models, such as patient-centered medical homes, are seeking to improve access to healthcare by allowing advanced practice providers, such as nurse practitioners, registered nurses, and physician assistants, to see patients under the overall supervision of physicians. A patient-centered medical home is a healthcare delivery model where healthcare services are coordinated through a primary care provider who seeks to ensure the patient has the necessary medical care at the appropriate time and location, and in a manner that the patient can understand.[2] Oregon was an early adopter of this model of care, and since 2011, has seen a "13% decline in emergency department visits, a 32% decline in hospital admissions for congestive heart failure, a 16% increase in primary care visits, and a 51% increase in the enrollment of patient-centered medical homes."[3]

While the patient-centered medical home model is gaining traction, one of the other significant advances in healthcare delivery is the utilization of telehealth. Telehealth encompasses "a broad variety of technologies and tactics to deliver virtual medical, health, and education services. Telehealth is not a particular service, but a collection of means to enhance care and education delivery."[4] Telehealth can include live video feeds between a patient and a doctor, forwarding electronic items to a provider, such as x-rays, photos, and medical records, remote patient monitoring, and treating patients through mobile health technologies such as cell phones, computers, and personal digital assistants.[4] As the lack of physicians in rural areas increases, telehealth remains a popular initiative to improve patient access to healthcare services. Kaiser Permanente implemented telehealth technologies, and from 2008 to 2013 saw an increase of 6.4 million virtual visits.[5]

Another goal of the various alignment models is to improve the coordination of a patient's healthcare services among multiple providers. In its simplest form, care coordination involves coordinating with a variety of healthcare providers to ensure that the patient receives the right care at the right time by the right person.[6] Under the fee-for-service reimbursement system, providers had no incentive to coordinate a patient's care, as the providers were paid the same regardless of whether that patient had positive health outcomes. In fact, while it was not the intention of most providers, they were paid more if the patient had an adverse result, as the basis of their payments was whether the procedure was medically necessary and whether the procedure was performed, not on the quality of the patient's care. However, because treatment of underlying conditions typically involves seeking care from a multitude of providers, and because the quality of the patient's overall care is factored into the final payment for the physician's services, it is vital that providers coordinate care to ensure that the patient receives high-quality care. This aspect is especially true in the primary care specialties, where coordination of care across the continuum is one of the major responsibilities of the primary care physician (PCP).

One of the big complaints clinicians have regarding care coordination is that the time spent coordinating a patient's care is often uncompensated, and as such, care coordination was lower on the totem pole than practicing medicine. For instance, during one patient's battle with liver cancer, a physician stated that during a particular 80-day period, there were "12 clinicians involved, 40 communications between Dr. Press [care coordinator] and other clinicians, 12 communications with the patient and/or his wife, 5 procedures, and 11 office visits."[7]

One way to increase coordination for healthcare services is for providers to form integrated practice units (IPU) or other clinical integrated networks (CINs).[8] "In an IPU, a dedicated team made up of both clinical and nonclinical personnel provides the full care cycle for the patient's condition. IPUs treat not only a disease but also the related conditions, complications, and circumstances that commonly occur along with it—such as kidney and eye disorders for patients with diabetes, or palliative care for those with metastatic cancer." Although the members of the networks may be located in many geographical areas and while the providers may specialize in many different areas of care, the members of the IPUs or CINs work as a team to treat the patient's condition.[8] For example, data have shown that an IPU that treats back pain has contributed to its patients missing four fewer days of work and requiring four fewer physical therapy visits.[8] IPUs can function as primary care teams; however, specialists are often required as well, since the range of patients' needs can be vast.[8]

Another way that alignment models can improve care coordination is through the use of electronic medical records. Electronic medical records ideally alert treating physicians when a patient has visited another provider. The patient's care coordinator can then follow up with the patient to better understand the patient's progression in treatment and also eliminate the possibility of the providing the patient with duplicative and unnecessary tests in the future.[9] Other processes assist in care coordination, such as assigning a team to communicate with the patient's primary care provider, tracking referrals to ensure that the patient is referred to providers that provide high-quality care, and providing a patient support system that understands the recovery process and why the patient is taking certain medications or being referred to a particular specialist.[10]

Another problem associated with the fee-for-service reimbursement system is that the delivery of healthcare services has often been centered on the provider as opposed to being focused on the patient. An example of provider-centered care is the Harris Hip Score often utilized by orthopedic surgeons. The Harris Hip Score requires patients to rate their pain, distance walked, and other activities after an orthopedic procedure.[11] The Harris Hip Score doesn't inquire about the quality or satisfaction of care the patients received while under the care of their particular provider.

Patient-centered care focuses on what matters to the patient. The Jefferson Scale of Patient's Perception of Physician Empathy is illustrative of patient-centered care attributes. This scale inquires about the physician's ability to understand the patients' emotions, whether the physician seems concerned about the patients and/or their families, whether the physician can see the problem from the patients' perspective, and whether the physician is an understanding physician.[12] It was found that this tool could predict positive and adverse patient outcomes, which were often not the case with the Harris Hip Score.[13]

Physicians who do not focus on patient-centered care can increase the likelihood of adverse health outcomes. For example, if a patient receives a mildly concerning test result from a provider with whom that patient does not have a personal relationship, the patient may ignore the test result; consequently, the mild condition could turn into a more serious condition. Further, physicians who practice provider-centric care are more likely to utilize "diagnostic tests, hospitalizations, prescriptions, and referrals among doctors who are poor communicators."[13]

Entities that value and implement patient-centered care respect the patients' needs and values, utilize care coordination and integration processes as well as information technology that educates the patients on their treatment and prognosis, and involve family and friends who provide emotional support to help alleviate the fear and anxiety of the treatment.[14]

Finally, in regards to quality improvements in value-based reimbursement, many models are seeking to reduce and/or eliminate the need to perform high-risk care that often results in injury and even death. As stated earlier, physicians until now have had no financial incentive to be concerned with a procedure's effect on a patient's overall safety, as they were financially rewarded for performing procedures regardless of the risk that procedure presented to the patient. However, under ACA and MACRA, providers must consider patient safety, as their payments will be negatively affected by an adverse medical event. Since the passage of the ACA and the transition toward value-based reimbursement, the U.S. Department of Health and Human Services estimates that preventable deaths and injuries have decreased by 15,000 and 560,000, respectively, which resulted in $4.1 billion in savings.[15]

Cost Improvements in the Value-Based Reimbursement Era

One of the central tenants of the ACA, MACRA, and value-based care is that healthcare costs must be reduced to provide value and allow the healthcare system in the United States to be more affordable. Value in the healthcare arena is defined as "health outcomes achieved per dollar spent,"[16] which requires healthcare organizations to reduce the costs of their care while also providing high-quality care. In reaching this goal, it is important for providers to decrease their utilization of expensive acute care and diagnostic tests.

A recent study found that providers make "approximately 12 million outpatient diagnostic errors each year."[17] Although some processes can be implemented that will reduce misdiagnosis and unnecessary tests, such as treatment checklists, the use of advanced health information technology (HIT) can be most beneficial. Common HIT systems can alert the physician that a test or order may be inappropriate for a particular ailment or that a particular test may be duplicative for that patient.[8] Further, these systems can recommend specific order sets as well as alert the provider regarding medication that may not be appropriate for the patient's diagnosis.[18]

Under the fee-for-service reimbursement system, utilization of acute care was high and vastly more expensive than physician office or clinical visits, as Figure 2.2.1 demonstrates[19]:

However, as stated previously, many healthcare providers are seeking to reduce the costs of their healthcare services, and as a result, the use of inpatient acute care services has declined by at least 6% since

Alternative Site of Care	Utilization	Commercial	Medicare
Emergency Room	5.6%	$1,595	$943
Urgent Care	45.8%	$116	$98
Physician Office Visits	30.9%	$98	$83
Other Clinics	5.4%	$57	$83
Do Nothing	0	0	0
Average Cost	100%	$176	$128

FIGURE 2.2.1 FFS Reimbursement for Utilization of Acute Care

2004.[20] Because of the declining utilization rates of diagnostic tests and acute inpatient care, advanced alignment models seek to promote the use of preventative care.

Traditionally, Medicare and commercial payers did not compensate preventative care, which typically includes tobacco cessation screening, alcohol abuse screening, and daily aspirin use, among other measures and activities. The payment for physician services was primarily reactionary to the disease or ailment instead of precautionary. However, with the passage of the ACA, compliant insurance plans must pay for up to nearly 20 preventative care counseling and screening measures for adults, as well as separate preventative care measures for women and children.[21] While Americans utilize preventative care measures at about one-half of the recommended rate, experts estimate that preventative care could prevent "the loss of more than two million life years annually."[22]

Another prevalent problem in the fee-for-service reimbursement environment was the duplication or provision of unnecessary care. Some providers may have duplicated tests because it was easier to re-perform the test rather than retrieve the results of the first test, or perhaps the duplicative test was conducted because the provider was financially incentivized to do so.[23] Other providers simply wanted to be as thorough as possible and would order various tests to confirm their diagnosis.[24] Providers can reduce the number of tests ordered by basing test administration on clinical need instead of ordering a battery of tests at once or ordering tests to confirm diagnoses. Also, as stated earlier, advanced HIT can reduce the number of unnecessary tests by using various prompts when a particular disease or ailment is identified.

The fee-for-service reimbursement system also resulted in long delays in access to healthcare services, which has both direct and indirect costs. In some markets, patients face week-long delays in accessing services and consequently do not keep their appointments, which can result in severe and dire consequences. Delays in access to care results in not only negative health outcomes, but also in lost revenue for the provider, as patients will seek providers whom they can sooner rather than later.[25]

Patient backlogs can be decreased by tracking patient appointments to determine trends that demonstrate when there is a surge in appointment requests, and modifying practice staffing and hours to accommodate the increase in appointment requests.[25] Additionally, healthcare providers should consider alternative methods of healthcare delivery, such as treating the patient through telemedicine, as previously discussed. Finally, the patient check-in process can be reduced or eliminated through the use of the online patient portal, where the patient can check in and complete the registration paperwork before the appointment.[26]

Under the fee-for-service reimbursement system, providers had no financial incentive to reduce serious complications from substandard medical care, other than those related to good public relations. In fact, a recent study found that treatment complications increased a hospital's profit margin. After looking at more than 34,000 inpatient surgical procedures, "Dr. Sunil Eappen of Harvard Medical School and his co-authors found that profit margins were 330% higher when privately insured patients suffered at least one complication. Among Medicare patients, profit margins were 190% higher."[27] The study found that hospitals stood to gain approximately $30,000 in additional revenue per complication.[27] However, under the payment reforms instituted by the ACA and MACRA, payments are reduced as more complications arise. Therefore, it is ever more important for organizations to increase the quality of their healthcare services.

In many situations, providers will have to design new processes of care to meet the challenges of achieving the now well-accepted Triple Aim of Healthcare Delivery: Patient Care, Population Health, and Cost Containment. Care process design will require providers to develop novel and innovative ways of delivering care, especially in the area of population health management.

While the scientific evidence base can inform this care design process, many of the questions that need to be answered have not been subjected to clinical trials and, therefore, the evidence base to support most of these new processes is sorely lacking. Therefore, those involved in the care design process will need to apply their knowledge, experience, and innovative ideas to the questions at hand to at least establish baseline guidelines that can then be continuously improved over time via an iterative process.

Coordinated and highly efficient care delivery across the care continuum will require input from many clinical and nonclinical disciplines. Their focus should be on the Care Process Unit (CPU), which is any commonly performed process or procedure with a clearly defined start and stop point. CPUs can be as simple as an office visit in a primary care clinic or as complex as a surgical procedure in a hospital operating room. Multidisciplinary care process design teams should be assembled around these CPUs, and the design process should be done in a nonhierarchical collaborative fashion that optimally should include patients to ensure the design of a patient-centered-care experience.

Providers' input will be essential. Hence, the process design system must be inclusive. Providers' contention that their patient population, practice location, facilities, staff, or equipment are unique also should be acknowledged, and care process design activities should be customized down to the individual provider, care team, and care location level.

Finally, design teams must recognize that care delivery no longer happens solely within the four walls of a traditional healthcare facility. Those providers who cannot utilize care processes within non-traditional settings, such as the community, home, or virtual environment (e.g., mobile technology, the Internet) will not be able to advance the Triple Aim.

Next Generation Alignment Models

One of the important ways to reduce costs and increase value is to form a patient-centered medical home. This model delivers care primarily through a patient's primary care physician and allows the patient to have care at the right time and place, and by the right person or facility.[28] "Care is facilitated by registries, information technology, health information exchange and other means to assure that patients get the indicated care when and where they need and want it in a culturally and linguistically appropriate manner."[28]

The patient-centered medical home has three levels, and becoming certified requires meeting varying standards in the following categories: providing enhanced access and continuity, identifying and managing patient populations, planning and managing care, providing self-care support and community resources, tracking and coordination of care, and measuring and improving performance.[29] Studies have shown that patient-centered medical homes reduce emergency room visits and costs, and improve patient outcomes, particularly in the areas of breast, cervical, and colorectal cancer.[30] Related to the patient-centered medical home is the specialty care medical home that is designed to treat patients with severe and chronic mental illnesses.

Whereas the patient-centered medical home focuses on providing care through a patient's primary care physician, the specialty care medical home seeks to provide care through a patient's specialty provider. Specialty care medical homes are geared more toward providing care to those suffering from severe and persistent diseases, such as cancer and schizophrenia.[31] Seeking care for these types of patients through a patient-centered medical home is not as effective since many primary care providers are not as experienced and knowledgeable in treating these diseases compared with specialists.[31]

One of the most popular forms of clinical integration is a clinically integrated network (CIN), or in the instance of payments issued by CMS, an accountable care organization. The CIN is a network of interdependent healthcare facilities and providers that work collaboratively to develop and sustain clinical initiatives. All participants (ideally, all types and forms of providers within a continuum of care) must commit to several key overarching tenets:

- They must adhere to evidence-based clinical protocols.
- They must ensure patient treatment information is readily available throughout the network.
- They must collaborate in the development of a prescribed set of quality and performance measures.
- They must agree to participate in the collection and sharing of data specifically related to their clinical performance and outcomes.

Also, the ability to participate within a payer contracting network is a fundamental prerequisite of being within the CIN. This performance will be evaluated by accepted standards, and participants must be willing to be subject to remediation directives (even sanctions and ultimately expulsion from the network) if their quality and performance standards are not up to par. Accountable care organizations are similar to CINs; however, ACOs often focus on Medicare patients.

CONCLUSION

The shift from fee-for-service reimbursement to value-based reimbursement has caused many healthcare providers to enter into a variety of transactions that give rise to the collaboration of multiple entities. This allows providers to provide healthcare services as a team instead of as individual providers. Examples of the newer and more advanced alignment models are medical homes, ACOs, and CINs. To take advantage of the reimbursement opportunities provided by the ACA and MACRA, many providers have developed numerous methodologies to increase the quality components of their care, such as participating in telemedicine and coordinating a patient's care through the use of care coordinators and electronic medical records. Providers have also been required to engage in cost-cutting tactics such as participating in bundled payment programs, developing and engaging in best practices that reduce the rate of medical errors, and cutting down on the utilization of inpatient admissions and unnecessary diagnostic testing. As the U.S. government continues its transformation to value-based reimbursement, the healthcare industry can expect to be required to continue developing other methods and practices that will increase quality while reducing cost.

REFERENCES

1. Access to health services. Healthypeople.gov. https://www.healthypeople.gov/2020/topics-objectives/topic/Access-to-Health-Services, citing Institute of Medicine, Committee on Monitoring Access to Personal Health Care Services. Access to health care in America. Millman M, editor. Washington, DC: National Academy Press; 1993. Accessed October 9, 2016.
2. What is the patient centered medical home? American College of Physicians. https://www.acponline.org/practice-resources/business/payment/models/pcmh/understanding/what-pcmh. Accessed October 9, 2016.
3. Sederstrom L. 7 ways to improve access. Modern Medicine Network. May 30, 2014. http://managedhealthcareexecutive.modernmedicine.com/managed-healthcare-

executive/content/tags/access-care/7-ways-improve-access?page=0,1. Accessed October 9, 2016.
4. What is Telehealth. Center for Connected Health Policy. http://cchpca.org/what-is-telehealth. Accessed October 9, 2016.
5. Sederstorm J. 7 ways to improve access. Modern Medicine Network. 3. May 30, 2014. http://managedhealthcareexecutive.modernmedicine.com/managed-healthcare-executive/content/tags/access-care/7-ways-improve-access?page=0,3. Accessed October 9, 2016.
6. The promise of care coordination: Transforming health care delivery. Families USA 4. April 2013. http://familiesusa.org/sites/default/files/product_documents/Care-Coordination.pdf.
7. WCOE: Challenges of care coordination in a fragmented health care system. National Coalition for Cancer Survivorship. August 22, 2014. https://www.canceradvocacy.org/news/challenges-of-care-coordination-in-a-fragmented-health-care-system. Accessed October 9, 2016.
8. Porter M and Lee T. The strategy that will fix health care. *Harvard Business Review*. October 2013. https://hbr.org/2013/10/the-strategy-that-will-fix-health-care
9. Improved care coordination: The need for better improved care coordination. Health IT. https://www.healthit.gov/providers-professionals/improved-care-coordination. Accessed October 9, 2016.
10. Royer R. *Transforming care coordination. H&HN Daily*. May 14, 2015. http://www.hhnmag.com/articles/3067-employees-raise-a-half-million-dollars-to-build-rural-replacement-building. Accessed October 10, 2016.
11. *Harris Hip Score*. Orthopaedic Scores. http://www.orthopaedicscore.com/scorepages/harris_hip_score.html. Accessed October 11, 2016.
12. Kane GC, Gotto JL, et. al. Jefferson Scale of Patient's Perceptions of Physician Empathy: Preliminary psychometric data. *Croat Med J*. 2007 Feb;48(1):81-86. https://www.ncbi.nlm.nih.gov/pmc/articles/PMC2080494/pdf/CroatMedJ_48_0081.pdf.
13. Rickert J Patient-centered care: What it means and how to get there. *Health Affairs Blog*. January 24, 2012. http://healthaffairs.org/blog/2012/01/24/patient-centered-care-what-it-means-and-how-to-get-there. Accessed October 11. 2016.
14. Shaller D. Patient-centered care: What does it take? Shaller Consulting 2-3. October 2007. http://www.commonwealthfund.org/usr_doc/Shaller_patient-centeredcare whatdoesittake_1067.pdf. Accessed October 11, 2016.
15. Corrigan JM, Wakeam E, et. al. Improved patient safety with value-based payment models. HFMA. https://www.hfma.org/Content.aspx?id=32499. Accessed October 11, 2016.
16. Porter M. What is value in health care? *N Engl J Med* 2010;363:2477-2481 ; Porter ME, Tesiberg EO, Redefining health care: creating value-based competition on results. Boson: *Harvard Business School Press*; 2006.
17. Fisher D. Accurate diagnosis: The conduit for value-based care. *Siemens Healthineers*. https://usa.healthcare.siemens.com/about-us/accurate-diagnosis-value-care. Accessed October 11, 2016.
18. Creating added value from clinical pathology laboratory testing produced improved outcomes at University of Mississippi Medical Center and Broward Health. *Dark*

Daily. June 22, 2015. http://www.darkdaily.com/creating-added-value-from-clinical-pathology-laboratory-testing-produced-improved-outcomes-at-university-of-mississippi-medical-center-and-broward-health622#axzz4MneGPDYF.

19. Yamamoto DH. Assessment of the feasibility and cost of replacing in-person care with acute care telehealth services. Barrington, IL: Red Quill Consulting, Inc. December 2014. http://www.connectwithcare.org/wp-content/uploads/2014/12/Medicare-Acute-Care-Telehealth-Feasibility.pdf. Accessed October 11, 2016.

20. Grube M, Kaufman K, et. al. Decline in utilization rates signals a change in the inpatient business model. *Health Affairs Blog.* March 8, 2013. http://healthaffairs.org/blog/2013/03/08/decline-in-utilization-rates-signals-a-change-in-the-inpatient-business-model. Accessed October 11, 2016.

21. Preventative care measures for adults. Healthcare.gov. https://www.healthcare.gov/preventive-care-adults. Accessed October 12, 2016.

22. Maciosek M, Coffield A, Flottemesch T, et. al. Greater use of preventative services in U.S. health care could save lives at little or no cost. *Health Affairs.* http://content.healthaffairs.org/content/29/9/1656.full. Accessed October 12, 2016.

23. Brenoff A. Medical tests: Study finds Medicare recipients are given too many unnecessary tests. *Huffington Post.* November 20, 2012. http://www.huffingtonpost.com/2012/11/20/medical-testing-medicare_n_2165461.html. Accessed October 12, 2016.

24. Colwell J. Reducing unnecessary testing. ACP Hospitalist. http://www.acphospitalist.org/archives/2011/07/coverstory.htm. Accessed October 12, 2016.

25. Trimming health care's excess waits and delays. Institute for Healthcare Improvement. http://www.ihi.org/resources/Pages/ImprovementStories/TrimmingHealthCaresExcessWaitsandDelays.aspx. Accessed October 13, 2016.

26. Weber S. Eleven ways to improve patient wait time. Physicians Practice 5. August 20, 2016. http://imaging.ubmmedica.com/all/editorial/physicianspractice/pdfs/Patient_Wait_Improvements.pdf. Accessed October 13, 2016.

27. Eappen S, Lane BH, et al. Relationship between occurrence of surgical complications and hospital finances. *JAMA.* 2013:309(15):1599-1606. http://jamanetwork.com/journals/jama/fullarticle/1679400. Accessed February 18, 2017.

28. What is the patient-centered medical home? American College of Physicians. https://www.acponline.org/practice-resources/business/payment/models/pcmh/understanding/what-pcmh. Accessed October 12, 2016.

29. Finger F. Is it worth it to become a patient-centered medical home. Medscape. October 22, 2013. http://www.medscape.com/viewarticle/812670. Accessed October 16, 2016.

30. Latest evidence: Benefits of the patient-centered medical home. NCQA. http://www.ncqa.org/programs/recognition/practices/pcmh-evidence. Accessed October 12, 2016.

31. Alakeson V, Frank R., and Katz R. Specialty care medical homes for people with severe, persistent mental disorders. *Health Affairs* 29(5):867-873. http://content.healthaffairs.org/content/29/5/867.full.pdf+html.

CHAPTER 3

Stage II Alignment Models and Entities

OVERVIEW OF STAGE II ALIGNMENT

The key to capitalizing on the shift to fee-for-value (FFV) compensation models and associated reimbursement structures lies within alignment models. The newer alignment structures vary significantly from previous alternatives, empowering physicians through a greater variety of integration strategies. As noted, these are considered Stage II alignment models and are the second step in the alignment structure, with Stage I being financial integration and Stage II being clinical integration. Stage II structures are increasingly focused on finding a "happy medium" between hospital and physician control as healthcare leaders realize the impact physicians, as the primary controllers of cost, can have on the success of an organization's participation in value-based reimbursement structures.

The clinical integration component of the Stage II alignment models is primarily the desire to create a collaborative and coordinated approach to healthcare delivery, while reliably producing high-quality clinical outcomes in the most cost-efficient manner possible. Essentially, the main emphasis of Stage II alignment models is to create value over volume, or achievement of the Triple Aim for healthcare. Thus, the key goals for clinically integrated organizations should be to (1) enhance patient experience of care, including access; (2) improve the overall management of health for a population; and (3) reduce or control the per-capita cost of care. Figure 2.3.1 identifies the benefits of clinical integration.

Patients/Community
- Access to high-quality, coordinated, and comprehensive care
- Potential for lower costs associated with healthcare services received

Providers
- Access to greater financial incentives
- Opportunity to drive healthcare quality and value
- Opportunity to engage in hospital-physician alignment

Hospitals
- Opportunity to cut costs and deliver improved patient-centric care
- Opportunity to engage in hospital-physician alignment

FIGURE 2.3.1 Benefits of Clinical Integration

The primary clinically integrated models prevalent in today's healthcare industry are quality collaboratives (QCs), patient-centered medical homes (PCMHs), clinically integrated networks (CINs), and accountable care organizations (ACOs). In the next sections, we will outline these models and their core tenets, as well as potential areas of concern.

CREATING LEGAL COMPLIANCE

A key benefit of achieving clinical integration is the ability to participate in certain practices that are otherwise deemed illegal by government regulations, such as joint negotiation of fees for services with payers. Thus, clinical integration must be established clearly based on the legal definition from the Federal Trade Commission (FTC). The FTC defines clinical integration as being "an active and ongoing program to evaluate and modify practice patterns by the network's physician participants and create a high degree of interdependence and cooperation among the physicians to control costs and ensure quality."

As noted above, one of the primary motivations for achieving clinical integration is to become eligible to participate in collective bargaining with payers for reimbursement of professional services rendered, which is is achievable by sharing significant financial risks among the providers or through clinical integration. To qualify as clinically integrated, the organization must achieve a few core components.

First, organizations should implement a standardized approach to care process design that emphasizes the use of evidence-based guidelines when available, and when not available, provides for the careful monitoring of outcome measures related to both cost and quality. Additionally, organizations should ensure that the providers are heavily invested in the success of the program, as they will drive the adoption of these principles and also determine the outcomes. Participating providers should be held accountable for the measurement, evaluation, and enforcement of their clinical outcomes and compliance with the standardized approach to care process design. This should include action on noncompliance and peer review functions to determine issues in quality.

Providers also should be expected to make meaningful contributions to the ongoing development and implementation of a standardized approach to care process design, including commitments of time, effort, data, and money. Finally, the network should develop a dedicated electronic platform by which participating providers can record and review data relating to cost, utilization, and quality of care, allowing efficient monitoring of performance.

Participating in joint contracting can lead to significant cost savings and increases in payer reimbursement. Organizations should not shy away from this option but they should consult third-party legal experts to ensure they are within FTC regulations.

STAGE II ALIGNMENT MODELS—CLINICAL INTEGRATION

Forming a clinically integrated organization will require significant collaboration among many different stakeholders and often among competitors. However, the right alignment strategy can increase collaboration among these distinct groups. Clinical integration can foster an organizational culture that supports teamwork and promotes an attitude for success and positivity, which are important, because without sufficient alignment and harmony among the practice partners, quality of care and population health management are likely to suffer. The alignment structures outlined in this section are the vehicles to achieve clinical integration. The following are brief overviews of the types of models available; we describe the structuring and implementation of these models more comprehensively in the next chapters.

Quality Collaboratives

While it is important to note the presence of QCs in the spectrum of contemporary alignment models, they usually are used as a stepping stone toward a more comprehensive clinical integration model. The general concept of a QC is a healthcare organization that has aligned itself with the focus of advancing the quality and efficiency of care delivery, including patient satisfaction. As with some of the other Stage II structures noted below, there are some accrediting bodies for QCs; however, many of them are self-appointed. QCs can be specific to an organization, a geographical location (i.e., a group of community physicians), or an individual service line within a hospital or health system. Again, because the sole priority of these models is achieving quality and efficiency for the organization, they can take multiple forms.

Organizations that have not fully altered their structure to align with value-based reimbursement find these programs appealing due to the low level of capital or time investment required. However, physicians are still expected to modify their thinking and focus on quality improvement. Thus, the outcome is an internal program that can be used to strategize for next steps, create a collaborative team of providers, and demonstrate to patients and payers a commitment to quality.

Alternatively, the relatively lax parameters create a system that can be somewhat forgotten or lowered on the list of priorities if more pressing matters present themselves. Moreover, these initiatives establish minimal cost accounting measures and do not necessarily incentivize providers to reduce their spending. Finally, participating organizations cannot engage in joint contracting with payers, as QCs do not meet the level of requirements needed to be considered clinically integrated.

Patient-Centered Medical Homes

PCMH is a new model that engages various types of providers (i.e., physicians, APPS, pharmacists, social workers, nutritionists, etc.) to develop lean process mapping, best-practice care design, time-driven activity-based cost accounting, and data-driven continuous process improvement to transform volume-based care processes and procedures into cost-efficient value-driven practices. This type of patient-centered care delivery affects everything from the way patients schedule appointments to the physical layout of the facility to the make-up of the multidisciplinary care teams. Essentially, the PCMH seeks to treat chronic health conditions through more effective primary care.

Although there is no single format for the formation of a PCMH, the National Committee for Quality Assurance (NCQA) is a general accrediting body that developed a voluntary recognition process in January 2008, with periodic updates under development and a revised list of criteria expected in March 2017. NCQA has proposed six separate standards with sub-elements listed for each for the PCMH 2017 requirements. The major standards would be

1. Team-Based Care and Practice Organization;
2. Knowing and Managing Your Patients;
3. Patient-Centered Access and Continuity;
4. Care Management and Support;
5. Care Coordination and Care Transitions; and
6. Performance Measurement and Quality Improvement.[1]

Organizations can achieve three "recognition levels" based on their score for the standards listed above. Again, those are just the criteria for being recognized as an NCQA PCMH; various other accrediting bodies exist as well.

The PCMH model is supported by various entities in the healthcare industry, including, but not limited to, payers (commercial and government), patients and physicians, and national policymakers. This support primarily stems from the fact that PCMH is one of the few clinical integration structures focused almost solely on the delivery of primary care, though many utilize primary care as the foundation. In its "Annual Review of Evidence 2014-2015" the Patient-Centered Primary Care Collaborative (PCPCC) reported that "55% of all medical office visits are for primary care, but only 4 to 7% of healthcare dollars are spent on primary care."[2] This statistic supports the theory that more focus should be placed on the delivery of primary care to control costs overall.

As noted above, PCMH models can improve coordination of care, access to care (both physically and virtually through established IT platforms), and patient outcomes, all while ensuring the best patient experience possible. However, it is not without some challenges—especially the ability of physicians to alter their methods of delivering care. This model also tends to work better for organizations that have transitioned to heavier volumes of value-based reimbursement contracts.

Finally, as with many of the clinical integration platforms, implementation will require significant capital and operating expenses due to investments in IT, leadership, staff, and even facility updates.

Clinically Integrated Networks

CINs are becoming increasingly common in the wake of the Accountable Care Era as organizations seek a systematic approach to high-value care delivery. CINs are formed with the intent of meeting all of the legal requirements for clinical integration as outlined above. The key components of CIN development are

- Measurement of outcomes (quality and cost);
- Use of outcomes to practice data-driven performance improvement;
- Establishment of a care management infrastructure;
- Implementation of a robust IT infrastructure; and
- Contracting for payer contracts on behalf of CIN members (usually with a heavy focus on value-based agreements).

Essentially, the goal of the first two components (i.e., establishing quality and cost measures and using the outcomes of such to determine areas of improvement) is seeking to respond to the expectations of population health management (PHM). PHM is the concept of monitoring the health outcomes for a specific population and moving toward a proactive delivery of care for a community. Again, the outcomes likely will lead to a focus on primary care development and the management of chronic conditions. Thus, CINs eventually should seek to establish a primary care base (though this is not necessary at the beginning).

This concept of value-based care has led to the transformation of care delivery methodology as noted in component three above. Coker utilizes the Care Process Design System (CPDS) to reform an organization's approach to the coordination of care through a complete overhaul of processes and protocols. It seeks to establish a continuum of care for an organization that relies on evidence-based, best-practice standards for all care delivery. It also uses a subset of physician leaders to drive these processes to instill a sense of responsibility and authority to these measures. Additionally, it relies on the use of certain IT requirements to analyze clinical data, assess health risks, monitor processes and procedures, and interact with a broader band of patients.

One of the most capital-intensive components of the CIN model is the establishment of an IT infrastructure that can support the other components. Thus, the CIN must have an electronic medical record (EMR) system that is accessible to all providers. Additionally, this EMR system should be able to share data with other platforms in order to increase the collaboration of care with other data repositories. Ideally, the IT system would also support significant analyses of cost data and areas of concern for supply and labor costs to maximize productivity. Finally, the system must be in full compliance with HIPAA privacy and security requirements.

Once all of the legal requirements for a clinically integrated organization have been met, the CIN can begin contracting on behalf of all participating providers and organizations. Due to the infrastructure established, these organizations likely will be more heavily involved in value-based reimbursement models such as shared savings agreements or bundled payments. The internal culture required to develop a CIN successfully will lead to financial success in these "at-risk" models, as quality and cost controls are vital components for all CINs.

There are various benefits to becoming involved in a CIN model, from both the organization's view and the physician's. It is one of the most efficient methods to align these parties in the delivery of high-value care. Additionally, it allows these entities to succeed under the value-based reimbursement paradigm. Finally, as noted, it permits providers and their organizations to participate in joint contracting efforts, which typically results in higher reimbursement.

CINs require significant capital and time expenditures on the part of all involved parties. However, if the capital is available, it is somewhat straightforward to coordinate the financial and administrative aspects of the collaboration, especially if an experienced contractor leads the effort. The true test is how well the CIN can become clinically integrated as various specialties and differing cultures are attempting to become a blended, coordinated unit of care. Thus, internal squabbles among the disparate providers and practices may occur.

Accountable Care Organizations

ACOs are "groups of doctors, hospitals, and other healthcare providers who come together voluntarily to give coordinated high-quality care to the Medicare patients they serve."[3] Essentially, ACOs are CINs that contract with Medicare for their services; thus, they are more highly regulated than CINs and fall under specific program models. Below, we briefly outline the primary ACO programs currently in effect with CMS.

1. *Medicare Shared Savings Program (MSSP):* The MSSP is an ACO model wherein the organization participates in a shared savings agreement with Medicare. This agreement can be one-sided risk (only participate in shared savings) or two-sided risk (participate in both shared savings and shared losses). Savings and losses are determined by calculating the difference of actual annual ACO expenditures for a defined population and a risk-adjusted benchmark for the projected expenditures.
2. *ACO Investment Model:* This model is an alternative to the MSSP model that utilizes prepaid shared savings to encourage organizations to participate in arrangements with greater financial risk. CMS is seeking to provide the infrastructure and capital for rural and underserved hospitals to take part in these models; thus, the ACO receives pay in advance for projected fixed and variable costs based on prospectively assigned beneficiaries.
3. *Advance Payment ACO Model:* The Advance Payment ACO model is similar to the ACO Investment model; however, the prepaid amounts are determined based on historically assigned beneficiaries.
4. *Next Generation ACO Model:* Next Generation ACO model participants typically are experienced ACOs that are interested in taking on more financial risk, and therefore reward, than their MSSP counterparts. Additionally, the outcomes of Next Generation ACO participants, such as quality and patient satisfaction, will be publicly reported.
5. *Pioneer ACO Model:* The Pioneer ACO model is for MSSP participants who, from the beginning of the MSSP, have been ready to participate in greater financial risk. Some participants have been able to move more quickly from the shared savings model toward PHM models; however, many others have dropped out of this Medicare program and have opted for models with lower risk.

ACOs have similar benefits as CINs; however, joint contracting will be solely for Medicare payments and reimbursement models. Moreover, patient benefits are limited to Medicare beneficiaries.

The ACO model is targeted toward participation in shared savings models and other structures that incentivize financial risk on behalf of the organization. While this option can have positive financial results for an organization, those that are not prepared to take on two-sided risk may struggle. Additionally, the quality metrics in Medicare ACOs are heavily weighted toward primary care delivery, which can make the allocation of shared savings difficult for specialty providers. Finally, patients can move into and out of the ACO at will; therefore, providers sometimes struggle to control patient quality and costs.

PHYSICIAN COMPENSATION FOR STAGE II ALIGNMENT STRUCTURES

Previously, we examined the effect value-based reimbursement models have had on the way physicians are compensated and incentivized. Specifically, there is an increased focus on incorporating incentives for quality and cost control across the spectrum of healthcare organizations. Stage II alignment structures are inherently more prepared to respond to these changes in compensation as their infrastructure is developed to support the measurement and improvement of these metrics. Moreover, as the result of value-based reimbursement, many organizations are eligible for shared savings, which can be distributed to the participating physicians. Therefore, Stage II alignment models are better equipped to support the allocation of these funds and justify these payouts from a fair market value standpoint.

As this shift requires significant infrastructure development and support (i.e., cost accounting and quality measurements), there is a clear case for making the transition as part of an overall strategic response to the Accountable Care Era. The organization should complete a "landscape review" of their current functions, described in detail below, and then determine how best to respond based on their particular organization. Because many of the core tenets of effectively creating a value-based compensation structure are encompassed in the development of a clinical integration strategy, it makes sense to pursue them as two parts of a whole strategy rather than as two separate tactics (this should also include the pursuit of value-based reimbursement models).

CONSIDERATIONS FOR STAGE II ALIGNMENT

The Accountable Care Era is ushering in a wave of challenges that pose unique challenges for organizations; however, with those challenges come opportunities to capitalize on the changes and develop an organization that not only responds to the needs of the physicians, but also provides a better patient experience. Organizations must review their current capabilities and gaps in infrastructure and resources to prepare and respond optimally to these changes. A few key considerations to take into account before deciding on a go-forward strategy are market conditions and reimbursement tactics, patient population and payer mix, and the breadth and depth of the provider network.

One of the primary factors to note before implementing a strategy is the market conditions of the organization's primary service area. Different markets are responding at different paces, and organizations should be wary of overreacting to these changes. For example, predominately fee-for-service markets do not necessarily require a complete overhaul of the existing systems; more importantly, the pursuit could be detrimental to the organization. Thus, organizations should consider more moderate strategies. Alternatively, organizations should not wait too long to develop a response strategy. Either way, some level of preparation is necessary for when the market does make the inevitable shift.

Additionally, organizations should understand their specific patient population and payer mix, especially as a prerequisite to pursuing an alignment or integration strategy. Practices with a strong mix of predominantly private payers have a higher bargaining power compared to their peers with a high mix of government payers. Moreover, a certain payer mix can help an organization decide which clinical integration initiative best fits its organizational structure, or whether one is necessary at all. For example, organizations with a higher percentage of CMS payments will be pressured to move toward value-based reimbursement models and subsequently clinically integrated structures. However, commercial payers are likely to catch up with CMS and eventually will become as aligned with value-based models as their government counterparts.

Finally, as is the case with most clinical strategies, the specific provider network should be considered before moving forward with any one alignment strategy. This is critical for clinical integration strategy for two primary reasons: (1) the physicians need to support the chosen initiative, and (2) certain clinical integration platforms require a primary care focus. The key to long-term sustainability of a clinically integrated network is having the support of the providers, as its success depends on the action of these physicians—both for quality and cost reasons. Meanwhile, certain Stage II alignment structures require a high volume of primary care physicians (i.e., PCMH models). Though, over the long-term, the incorporation of primary care likely will be necessary for all models.

CONCLUSION

There is a multitude of strategies for transitioning from a "fee-for-service" to a "fee-for-value" structure; however, all rely on the understanding that this shift is inevitable and approaching rapidly in some areas. Again, while this may seem intimidating to some organizations, there are significant opportunities on the horizon for everyone who is willing to recognize their current capabilities and adapt to these changes. The ultimate goal is to develop a viable strategy that incorporates aspects of traditional and contemporary alignment to meet the needs of the shifting healthcare landscape.

In the next few chapters, we will review how these Stage II alignment models can be formed and implemented so as to realize the highest levels of efficiency and cost benefits for an organization. However, it is important to note that clinical integration is not always the answer; rather, all of this should be considered as one potential response to the value-based paradigm shift. On the other hand, clinical integration efforts can prepare organizations to respond to the other demands of this new FFV industry.

REFERENCES

1. PCMH 2017 Recommendations Table. NCQA. http://www.ncqa.org/Portals/0/PublicComment/PCMH%202017%20Recommendations%20Table.pdf?ver=2016-06-13-094129-053. Accessed November 8, 2016.
2. Nielsen M, Buelt L, Patel K, and Nichols L. The patient-centered medical home's impact on cost and quality, review of evidence, 2014-2015. Patient-Centered Primary Care Collaborative. Accessed November 8, 2016.

3. Centers for Medicare & Medicaid Services. Accountable care organizations (ACOs): General information. CMS.gov. https://innovation.cms.gov/initiatives/ACO. Accessed November 8, 2016.

SECTION 2

CHAPTER 4

Structuring Stage II Alignment Models

In Chapter 3 of Section 2, we reviewed the concept of Stage II alignment models and the common forms that they take. In the next two chapters, we will focus on the methods of developing and implementing a CIN, as it makes State II alignment models somewhat easier to understand. These same foundations are similar across all Stage II alignment models and can be used to begin working in that direction. However, if an organization wishes to pursue a foundation that is not a CIN, it must be aware of some differing legal and structural concerns. The establishment of another model calls for additional research or the utilization of a third-party legal expert.

Although we previously addressed the topic of necessary infrastructure and legal considerations, we will delve into more detail in this chapter. The core purpose of all of these requirements is to maintain the patient-centric aspect of the CIN while considering ways to reduce costs and improve the quality of care. All other infrastructure considerations are merely methods to support the Triple Aim. Key factors when establishing a clinically integrated organization include:

- Defining clearly the goals and objectives of the entity (these may evolve and, in fact, mature over time, particularly if the CIN initially is formed on a much more limited scale, perhaps through an IPA or PHO);
- Utilizing resources that are currently available within the organizational consortium to build the CIN;
- Emphasizing the utilization of a physician-driven model;
- Designing a program that meets the consumer healthcare needs of the service area of the CIN;

- Initiating the process with modest clinical metrics and then maturing them as the process and CIN develop with both experience and success;
- Establishing clinical protocols that cover an extensive continuum of care, including inpatient, outpatient/ambulatory, home care, skilled nursing facilities, and hospice/palliative care;
- Committing to an investment in a sufficient infrastructure (primarily an IT infrastructure) that electronically measures performance, compares against benchmarks, and targets improvements needed; and
- Establishing effective communication among the providers, employers, and other participants, including third-party payer contractors.

Possible Structures for the CIN

Before we move into the infrastructural components of the CIN, it is important to note that there are a few possible arrangements for these CINs to take as it pertains to how the entity is formed initially and what primary body is driving the development. The Federal Trade Commission (FTC) has allowed CINs to form by permitting primarily hospitals and physicians to align through integration. This authorization has also enabled them to negotiate collectively without being subject to antitrust violations, assuming certain criteria are met. This makes forming a CIN paramount from a good business plan perspective (i.e., structured in such a way that the CIN has the greatest likelihood of performance and financial success), and also as a means to ensure its structure is within the safe harbors of antitrust legislation.

IPA-Directed CIN

Chapter 1 of this section presented IPAs as a type of Stage I alignment model. To review, an IPA essentially is a grouping of independent physician practices with hospitals/health systems, along with their employed physicians often participating as members also. In this instance, the IPA (again, led by physicians) would take the leadership role of the CIN, possibly with allied healthcare providers included. Often, since IPAs are physician-led, hospitals and other healthcare providers assume a subordinate position. Hospitals could be a primary partner in forming the IPA. Thus, the leadership presumption position of the IPA being led by physicians may change. This model would also consider a PCMH structure as a part of the foundation of the CIN operation.

Multispecialty Group-Directed CIN

A multispecialty physician group, usually one that is quite large and has a broad cross-section of representation of both primary care and specialists, could be the leader of the developing CIN. In such an example, the CIN (led by the multispecialty group) may approach a hospital or health system to contract for inpatient services.

The PHO-Directed CIN

The PHO-directed CIN adopts a more traditional physician-hospital organization at the center of the CIN. The PHO creates the working relationships with both physician practices and a hospital system, generally with the hospital taking the leadership role in its development and, often, the capitalization.

Integrated Delivery Network-Directed CIN

This model places the consortium of integrated delivery network providers at the center of the involvement and "ownership" of the CIN. As such, the integrated delivery network may employ and/or contract with its physicians and, typically, it is led by a health system/hospital.

Payer-Directed CIN

This model focuses on a private payer's formation of a direct partnership with physicians, creating a physician-only CIN that would subcontract for hospital/health system services. This CIN construction could also be between IPAs and/or PHOs or multispecialty group models. The intent is for the private payer to be the partner that provides needed financial support for infrastructure development, including IT, data aggregation, and overall assimilation of the CIN's operations. It could contract with hospitals/health systems and even individual ancillary service providers that would be the conduit for the full continuum of healthcare delivery services.

Joint Venture Structures

CINs can be assembled through joint venture structures. CMS requires a Medicare ACO to have a formal legal structure that allows that organization to receive and distribute the payments for shared savings to participating providers. Even within a joint venture scenario, private CINs have to be concerned about antitrust and how best to form these entities legally. Examples of certain joint venture opportunities include the following:

- An existing integrated delivery network affiliating through a joint venture and/or a merger with another health system or hospital and/or an existing CIN;
- A primary care medical home practice combining with a multi-specialty group practice; or
- A CIN merging with one or more medical homes and multispecialty group practices.

These affiliations can be combined in a variety of ways, as long as they are appropriately structured to respond to antitrust considerations.

LEGAL CONSIDERATIONS

As noted above, the formation and operation of a CIN relies on a number of components in its legal structure and may take many forms. A CIN can be in the form of a joint venture and sponsored by payers, other integrated systems, PHOs, multi- or single-specialty groups, IPAs, as well as hospitals.

Participation Agreements

Each of these legal structures will require legal documentation to support its particular structure and purposes. All of these organizations, regardless of form, will need to obtain a commitment from the physicians who are part of the organization to participate in its activities and its operations. Specifically, each physician will need to agree to perform in ways that are required for the CIN to achieve clinical and financial integration. Additionally, the physicians will need to perform in a manner that is consistent with the payment systems that are involved. The agreements between physicians and CINs are called "Participation Agreements."

The physicians' Participation Agreement is the legal document that engages the physicians in the business enterprise of the CIN and commits them to support its business purposes. Creating the

Participation Agreement between the physician and the CIN calls for consideration of several factors. The form of the Participation Agreement will be customized to the arrangement.

The contents of Participation Agreements must include a sufficient commitment from the physicians to pass antitrust muster. The physicians must commit to being sufficiently integrated on either a clinical basis or a financial basis. The FTC has published "safety zones" that give guidance and meaning to the terms clinical integration and financial integration.

Physician Participation Agreements live in the narrow intersection of five different legal and regulatory regimes. The laws involved include the Stark law, the Anti-Kickback Statute, federal tax exemption laws, antitrust laws, and state insurance laws. The regulatory bodies enforcing these laws include CMS, the IRS, the FTC, the Department of Justice (DOJ), and state insurance regulators. Because many laws and regulatory bodies affect the Participation Agreements, it is necessary to include contractual provisions that address some core specification of all of these laws to be compliant. Additionally, these same laws present a series of options or opportunities for different contractual provisions that optionally may be a part of a Participation Agreement.

If an organization decides to become a Medicare ACO, it is possible to obtain waivers[1] from applicability of the Stark law, the Anti-Kickback Statute, the antitrust laws, and from concerns about an organization's tax-exempt status. These waivers are "self-implementing," meaning that properly structured Medicare ACOs do not need to file applications for waivers, but may proceed with their business with a degree of comfort that they would be exempt from a challenge if they establish proper policies and procedures. In contrast, CINs that are not Medicare ACOs do not enjoy the benefit of the waivers and must structure their arrangements in ways that are compliant. Also, they must consider whether to seek specific private letter rulings or other forms of regulatory approval that will allow them to operate their business successfully.

Antitrust

Most physicians and hospitals in a geographic market typically would be considered to be competitors. If they join in an unbridled effort to raise prices, that is a violation of the antitrust law and would be viewed as collusion. They could also attempt to reduce the quality or volume of care that is delivered or reduce competition, all of which would be considered as harmful to the marketplace. Accordingly, the effect that a CIN or ACO has on the marketplace is an important consideration from the antitrust perspective. The FTC would weigh the relative benefits and efficiencies delivered by an ACO or CIN and balance that against the anti-competitive effects that would be seen as being harmful to the consumer or the marketplace.

The FTC's antitrust safety zones for healthcare indicate that organizations will be safe from an antitrust challenge if they achieve sufficient "clinical integration" and/or "financial integration." Financial integration may include initial investments, annual dues, incentive payments, withholds, and shared risk, which may take many forms. Clinical integration involves aligning medical practice activities with quality of performance, outcomes, and value. Both clinical and financial integration typically will demonstrate efficiencies, and both usually will require an actual investment of both human and financial capital by all parties.

To avoid an antitrust challenge, CINs should evaluate and modify practice patterns. They must create interdependence among physicians to help control costs and to help ensure quality. It will be vital for CINs to monitor and control utilization. Additionally, although it can be a controversial subject, CINs should be selective in choosing physicians who are genuinely interested in focusing on efficiencies and enhancing the delivery of quality care in their market.

Antitrust concerns will arise if the CIN inappropriately shares competitively sensitive information among its participants or if those involved to collude in their provision of healthcare. Also, participants in a CIN should be careful about providing or creating any links between their activities in the CIN and other activities in which they may engage, as these connections generally are suspect.

To avoid or minimize these concerns, CINs should focus first on achieving clinical integration and then pursue financial integration. Reversing this sequence can lead to greater scrutiny from regulators, chiefly the FTC.

The Anti-Kickback Statute

The Anti-Kickback Statute (AKS) prohibits knowing or willful payments or any inducement in return for referrals. Therefore, to avoid being attacked for a violation of the AKS, it is necessary for the CIN to ensure that payments are not made with the intent to induce referrals nor with the intent to limit medically necessary services for patients. Thankfully, safe harbors are available.[2] The safe harbor that is used most often is known as the "personal services and the management contracts" safe harbor. This regulation requires that the physician Participation Agreement meet seven standards:

1. The agreement must be in writing;
2. The agreement must describe all of the services to be provided;
3. If the agreement is periodic, sporadic, or part-time, it must specify exactly the schedule of the intervals;
4. The agreement must be for not less than one year;
5. Compensation must be set in advance, consistent with fair market value and not determined in a manner that takes into account the volume or value of referrals;
6. It cannot involve the counseling or promotion of a business that violates state or federal law; and
7. The aggregate services must not exceed those reasonably necessary to accomplish the commercially reasonable purposes of the agreement.

When parties enter into these agreements, determining what is set in advance, fair market value, and commercially reasonable are the most challenging aspects of the accords. Typically, CINs will engage a third-party valuation organization to review and comment on the terms of the Participation Agreements and the distribution structure of the CIN to ensure that the agreement is properly set in advance, at fair market value, and commercially reasonable.

Stark Law

The Stark law prohibits a physician from making referrals for certain designated health services (DHS) payable by Medicare to an entity with which he or she (or an immediate family member) has a financial relationship (ownership, investment, or compensation), unless an exception applies. Unlike the AKS, Stark is a strict-liability statute. The Anti-Kickback Statute requires that a provider commit a willful or intentional act to violate the AKS, whereas with Stark, the intent of the provider is not determinative of whether a violation occurs.

Participation Agreements may fit into any one of several Stark law exceptions, including bona fide employment, physician services, personal services arrangements, physician recruitment and retention, isolated transactions, and risk-sharing arrangements. The parties must carefully analyze the specifics of the CIN Participation Agreement to identify the correct Stark law exception that they will use. To meet these exceptions, the CIN Participation Agreement must be structured to include provisions that are similar to the requirements of the AKS safe harbor. Stark law exceptions normally require a written agreement of one year or more that does not vary compensation based on the volume or value of referrals, and the compensation must be set in advance, be commercially reasonable, and set within fair market value limits. Again, this is a zero-tolerance statute; i.e., the law must be met or it will result in a violation.

Tax Exemption

If a tax-exempt hospital is involved in the CIN, steps must be taken to ensure the protection of the hospital's tax-exempt status. No hospital will be willing to put its tax exemption at risk in the formation of a CIN. Under Internal Revenue Code Section 501(c)(3), it is prohibited to have inurement or private benefit to individuals associated with the CIN. This prohibition affects all compensation arrangements between hospitals and physicians, including those of a CIN that involves a hospital. Similar to Stark and Anti-Kickback, payments that are commercially reasonable and consistent with fair market value are typically viewed as being acceptable. Again, it is necessary to obtain a third-party opinion of the arrangement to be sure that it is appropriate.

To further enhance the protection against IRS challenge, the CIN should avoid entering into unrelated businesses that would generate taxable unrelated business income. If the hospital is a major sponsor or owner of the CIN, it will also be necessary to include provisions in the documentation that recite that the CIN's principal purpose is consistent with the charitable mission of the tax-exempt hospital.

State Insurance Law

State insurance laws regulate organizations that accept some form of financial risk for the delivery of healthcare. Additionally, the risk that has been accepted has to be the risk associated with other parties, not for itself. For example, if a hospital accepts capitation from a payer, and the hospital's capitation covers only goods and services delivered by the hospital, that position is not viewed as an insurance risk. However, if the hospital accepts a capitation payment for its own goods and services and those of other participants in the CIN (such as physicians), that in many states will be viewed as an insurance risk that is subject to state regulation.

Although there have been a variety of attempts to make insurance regulation at least somewhat uniform, the fact remains that the United States is a crazy quilt of 50 different sets of laws. Accordingly, when the CIN is being established, if any form of financial risk is being accepted, the CIN will need to evaluate whether the risk-bearing arrangement is one that is covered by state insurance laws. If it is, the organization will need to take steps to obtain regulatory approval, licensure, and possibly qualification as a health insuring corporation with appropriate financial reserves.

In summary, the creation of a CIN involves not only the formation of a legal entity and the execution of Participation Agreements, but also includes compliance with at least five significant laws and regulations and regulatory regimes. Proper planning and preparation for meeting these regulatory requirements is necessary to avoid unwelcome surprises.

FINANCIAL CONSIDERATIONS

As with any formation of a new business model, numerous financial considerations must be made before entering into a binding agreement. These range from how best to fund the initiative and require financial risk from all participants to how best to allocate the shared savings achieved. As with most of the foundational components, there are varying methods for achieving financial integration and compliance while developing a thriving entity. Thus, it is important to consult a third-party expert or complete comprehensive research on all of these matters.

Allocation of Start-Up Costs and Physician Input

Based on the models for a CIN as outlined above, the funding for start-up costs could emerge in a variety of ways (i.e., from the hospital, fees from participating providers, etc.). The key is to ensure that these start-up costs are adequately repaid before distributing shared savings to the participating physicians so as not to give the impression the funding was in any way a handout. It is still possible for the hospital to loan these funds to the CIN, with the CIN repaying the hospital via the shared savings. Alternatively, if a group of practices or other provider organizations align to create the CIN, the separate entities could put up these start-up costs (assuming that physicians are partners in the practices), as this implies that the physicians are still taking on the risk and therefore can substantiate the return of shared savings. If certain physicians are not partners of the practice, the portion of physicians who invested in the CIN, or the practice itself, would need to be reimbursed before the other physicians receive shared savings.

These start-up costs can entail a variety of expenses, all related to the development and implementation of a CIN. For example, the costs could include consulting and legal advisory services, infrastructure development (i.e., IT and care management), staffing improvements, facilities expansions, and marketing activities. Again, all of this should be considered before the engagement to determine the priorities of these developments and the required start-up costs from each entity.

Additionally, due to the legal aspects of the CIN, many advisors will encourage financial commitment from the participating physicians to pass antitrust muster, though this is not a requirement. Again, clinical integration can be equally compelling; however, the financial commitment is a clear indication that physicians are invested in the model and, therefore, deserve remuneration for their efforts. As such, the FTC has published "safety zones" that give guidance and meaning to the terms clinical integration and financial integration.

A common way to not only fund start-up costs but also ensure financial commitment to the CIN is to charge an entry fee to physicians who wish to enter into the organization. A conservative reading of the FTC safety zone suggests that paying a fee is helpful in that it indicates that financial integration exists among the participating providers. However, charging a fee is not mandatory. To encourage physicians to participate and to help all physicians feel like they are equals, many CINs do not charge an entry fee to the participating providers. As noted, other CINs need capital to pay for information technology and other business resources that are necessary to their operations. By charging a large number of physicians a modest fee, the CIN can accumulate a substantial amount of capital that will help pay for its business infrastructure. Some CINs have begun charging annual dues or maintenance fees.

Some CINs are owned entirely or in part by physicians. In these ownership situations, it is necessary for the participating physicians to purchase their ownership interest. Please note that purchasing an ownership interest in a CIN differs from paying a fee to be a participating provider. A securities offering usually will be necessary to establish any ownership arrangement of this type.

Compensation Methodologies

As we will discuss below with the allocation of expenses, some CINs do not provide direct compensation to physicians; rather, they allocate shared savings. This decision largely depends on how the revenue is determined (i.e., as a single entity or as separate, collaborating entities) and whether the practices continue to operate independently in some fashion. Either way, the CIN still can contract on behalf of the practices, though it may determine if that is done as a conglomerate of practices or a singular NewCo.

CINs are moving toward a fee-for-value compensation paradigm along with all other organizations; however, these Stage II alignment models are creating more of a focus on these initiatives. Productivity will remain important in that physicians will need to produce enough to meet volume requirements for overhead and related costs. However, going forward, quality of care and evidence-based results will become more of a focal point. Thus, it is important to understand the types of compensation models CINs are using.

Two payment methodologies cover the spectrum of clinical integration compensation. First are the physician-specific models, which utilize payments such as fee-for-service, management revenue, and performance-based payments. While a CIN negotiates with the payers for its member's services, fee-for-service payments received from payers may be distributed to participating providers in amounts reflecting the amount of payments received by the network with respect to the provision of service by such participating providers. Medical management or consulting fees received from payers may be distributed to participating providers on a per-member-per-month basis consistent with the amounts received by the CIN. In addition, payments based on the performance of quality measures, outcomes, and value, like gain sharing, shared savings, bundled payments, and similar payments received from payers by the network, may be distributed to participating providers consistent with their performance under such programs (as will be discussed in more detail, below).

Group participation serves as the second incentive methodology for the clinically integrated network. Similar to the individual physician method, the group participation method has overhead and reserves/ROI expenses. However, the revenue in the group participation model has no individual component. Similar to the individual physician model previously described, multiple types of revenue (fee-for-service, management, quality, and CIN funding) could be negotiated by the CIN. The key difference is that in the group participation model, the revenue generated is consolidated by the CIN, and then after the deduction of the mentioned expenses, a pool of funds is available for distribution to the CIN physicians.

Distribution of Expenses

Similar to the concept of start-up costs, the payment of expenditures incurred by the CIN is somewhat dependent on the structure of the organization. If the CIN can accrue a level of shared savings that is sufficient to cover the expenses of the CIN, it is best practice to have those expenses paid directly from that fund before the CIN makes distribution payments to the physicians.

Alternatively, if the CIN is incurring costs at a rate higher than the shared savings gained, the CIN will have to utilize the physicians or organizations to pay back these expenses. Again, if the hospital or practice(s) fund these expenses, the primary goal, once shared savings are achieved, should be to reimburse those entities for their contributions.

The types of costs depend on how the organization is established. For example, a practice could be a participant of the CIN, but all individual practice expenses could be considered on an independent basis (i.e., practices divide expenses incurred on behalf of the CIN as opposed to those incurred on behalf of their individual practice). In that scenario, it is likely that the CIN is participating in "one-offs" engagements, such as bundled payments or other reimbursement methods. Thus, any other expenses or revenues made outside that arrangement would be kept on the individual level. On the other hand, the CIN could become the new company for all procedures being done by the involved parties. In that scenario, the CIN would accrue all revenue on behalf of all practices and then handle all expenses. Essentially, it is determined by how integrated the entities are (even if they are technically clinically integrated in some capacity).

Shared Savings Distribution Model

A primary intended outcome for CINs is to develop a pool of shared savings that provides a benefit to the payers, creates a fund to reimburse parties and continue to build infrastructure, and serves as a method to reward the physicians for their efforts. Once the CIN has accounted for the three components listed above (i.e., repayment of start-up costs/loans, overhead expenses, and physician compensation), the remaining shared savings can be distributed to participating physicians.

Each organization can determine the most efficient and fair manner to distribute shared savings; however, it is important that the considerations noted in start-up costs are taken into account (i.e., the hospital should be repaid for loans to the CIN). Furthermore, it is likely that these arrangements will continue to evolve and mature in concert with the organization itself. As with all incentive and compensation programs, these shared savings are subject to fair market value and commercial reasonableness determinations.

While these have been considerations within healthcare transactions for many years, the concept of pay-for-performance compensation programs in the context of CINS, ACOs, or other Stage II alignment models is relatively new and, therefore, has limited historical precedent as it relates to determining FMV and commercial reasonableness for such transactions. Unlike traditional physician compensation arrangements, there are no independent industry surveys that provide an overall indication of market conditions, incentive compensation structures and associated payouts, and other related benchmarks. Further, given the variability in focus and composition of these arrangements, any market data would be difficult to use/apply at best.

Indeed, there is no single industry-wide approach to valuing shared savings incentive programs. In our view, valuation of such programs should focus chiefly on the structure of the arrangement and the variables that impact what may be paid out to participating physicians. Primarily, the organization should determine if the structure makes sense and whether there is a reasonable relationship between the distributions to the physicians and the contributions made by the physicians to the generation of the shared savings.

This concept is highlighted in the IRS Service Fact Sheet with respect to guidance for tax-exempt organizations participating in the MSSP. Obviously, not all organizations will be subject to the MSSP regulations, although the guidance is still worthwhile when evaluating similar types of programs. Specifically, the Fact Sheet notes the following:

> *The tax-exempt organization's share of economic benefits derived from the ACO (including its share of Shared Savings payments) is proportional to the benefits or contributions the tax-exempt organization provides to the ACO. If the tax-exempt organization receives an ownership interest in the ACO, the ownership interest received is proportional and equal in value to its capital contributions to the ACO and all ACO returns of capital, allocations and distributions are made in proportion to ownership interests.*[3]

In addition to the format by which these payments are made, it is important that there are incentives that align with the goals of quality improvement, cost reduction, care coordination, and patient experience. In short, the initiative set forth for the CIN should seek to reduce costs for the overall organization while maintaining quality and patient satisfaction scores. These shared clinical integration goals could take various forms; however, a common group goal is the management of chronic illnesses such as:

- Diabetes
- Coronary artery disease
- Heart failure
- COPD
- Hypertension
- Asthma

Once the CIN can determine total shared savings and achievement of targeted performance levels with respect to quality and satisfaction measures, it likely is justified to distribute some payments. However, it is important that the CIN take precautions, especially in the first few years of the arrangement, to ensure that these savings are attributable to the functions of the CIN and sustainable in the long-run.

As noted, the primary concern is whether the distribution payments to the physicians will correspond with the effort expended, as well as the start-up costs incurred. However, we again emphasize the need for an external or internal audit of these payments as it pertains to the legal and regulatory requirements.

OPERATIONAL CONSIDERATIONS

A number of items fall under the umbrella of operational considerations, including the alignment of organizational goals, development of clinical pathways and protocols, implementation of sufficient IT infrastructure, and determination of oversight and governance structures. All of these factors will be the key to determine how well the CIN clinically integrates, as opposed to stopping at financial and legal integration. These issues will be the keys to developing a long-term, sustainable CIN. Moreover, their achievement is what makes the CIN legally compliant, which underscores the need to attend to and not ignore their importance.

Alignment of Organizational Goals

The first step to attaining organizational goals is to begin with the end in mind. Where are we trying to go and who can help us get there? Leaders of the CIN must identify the goals through a structured process that involves all of the stakeholders in their development. This process creates buy-in for the participants and provides practical and attainable objectives that reflect the reality that frontline healthcare professionals face. Moreover, it seeks to establish a culture that focuses on quality, patient experience, organizational performance, and efficiencies in care.

The next step is to refine the goals so they can be monitored and measured to ensure progress. Additionally, an incentive system needs to be instituted that will recognize progress in achieving the goals and reward the clinical and administrative staff and management who put forth the effort in achieving the objective.

Finally, organizational strategic goals must be reexamined periodically to ensure they remain relevant in the ever-changing healthcare context. As time passes and the organization develops, new goals will emerge to replace old ones, and the process will repeat itself. An organization also can raise the bar and use previously achieved goals as a baseline for future improvement.

Development of Clinical Pathways and Protocols

A primary goal should be to establish a systematic approach to improving care delivery, especially given the participation in shared savings arrangements or bundled payments. It becomes much easier to control costs, increase efficiencies, and maintain quality if the entire organization is functioning in a similar manner. Thus, organizations should consider a function for designing evidence-based care processes and procedures and implementing those effectively. Physicians tend to balk at the concept of an organization dictating the way they deliver care; however, the intent of this initiative is not to take away the autonomy or decisions of a physician, but to set a standardized approach to process and procedure improvement.

As part of this CPDS (described in the previous chapter), it is necessary for an individual or group of people to review quality outcomes and cost accounting measures on an ongoing basis. Feedback loop mechanisms should be created to facilitate the continuous value-generation. Moreover, the organization should have policies and procedures in place that hold physicians accountable for all instituted quality, satisfaction, and cost measures to justify the distribution of shared savings, if applicable.

Implementation of Sufficient IT Infrastructure

Another immediate need for all CINs is a robust IT infrastructure. This topic was discussed briefly in the previous chapter, noting specifically the need for an EMR that at the very least is able to interface with the others in the CIN. This interface presents a challenge to most organizations, as many EMRs are not built to allow the sharing of data across systems. Nevertheless, this capability is the bare minimum for a CIN to function and is a requirement.

Eventually, the goal is for all physicians to integrate into a single data repository that can report on quality requirements and serves as a patient communication and outreach system, functioning as a health information exchange or HIE. The system should be able to support the growth of the CIN as it expands to incorporate other physicians and specialties.

There is a significant need for CINs to invest in a cost accounting system. This system should not only determine the true supply costs for the procedures (i.e., use of machinery, drugs and medical instruments, implants, etc.) but also the associated labor costs. Thus, the system should be able to measure time spent in the OR, turnover time, etc. While this may seem to be a daunting task, there are organizations that are completing these processes, which will be critical in participating in value-based reimbursement models.

As part of the IT infrastructure, the CIN also needs to consider how billing and collections will be completed on behalf of the CIN. As noted, billing processes will no longer be as straightforward as reporting procedures and service invoicing. Going forward, it will require accurate reporting of achievement of quality and cost metrics to effectively determine reimbursements under a fee-for-value model.

Oversight and Governance

While oversight and governance may not seem as critical as the other considerations discussed, it can be a major point of tension for CINs as previously disparate physicians seek to establish a new hierarchy and structure. Further, this structure likely will bring forth any underlying concerns between the hospitals and practices and between the different specialties, as well.

The governance structure pursued need to be able to support the demands of the CIN, including those imposed by regulatory bodies. It should demonstrate a process that achieves the following:
- Development and approval of care processes (a standardized and systematic approach to care process/procedure improvement—not the application of standardized methods, techniques, technology, supplies or equipment at the frontline care delivery level);
- Development of measures that identify high-quality, low-cost providers who can be used to determine "best practices" within the CIN;
- Benchmarking of individual and group performance against competitors and established standards of care;

- Education geared at the promotion of care process improvement and value-based care delivery; and
- Utilization of a referral-optimization system within the CIN to ensure the optimal match of patient needs with care provider capabilities and the simultaneous improvement in individual physician/surgeon performance.

Thus, we recommend that as part of the definitive agreements for the CIN, a specific governance structure is outlined that includes a hierarchy of multidisciplinary management members who work in concert to achieve the tenets of clinical integration and the above objectives.

CONCLUSION

In this chapter, we have outlined the key considerations for the formation of a CIN; however, establishing an ACO, PCMH, or QC would require essentially the same tenets (though they may be tweaked slightly). Either way, this information should offer a roadmap for all of the concepts an organization should consider before moving forward with any of these arrangements. It is important to note that these structures can be extremely time and capital intensive; however, the outcomes can be an organization that is primed to capitalize on the shift to value-based care.

Moreover, any one of these tenets alone could be a beneficial concept to consider for an organization (e.g., development of evidence-based, clinical care processes and procedures). Again, it is important for an organization to consider all of its alternatives in responding to this shift in the industry and not overreact or impulsively become involved in one of these initiatives. Organizations must begin making some movement toward preparing for these changes, as they are inevitable.

In all of these areas, we urge organizations to complete additional research, specifically in areas where there may be a gap in addressing this structure. If additional help is still required or desired, there are various third-party options that can assist you in reviewing these considerations and determining the best go-forward strategy, as well as analyzing the projected cost for implementing these.

REFERENCES

1. Note that the waivers only apply to ACOs, not CINs. Additionally, the waivers do not prevent the individual states from prosecuting healthcare fraud related to kickback and state-based Stark laws.
2. It is important to note that safe harbors apply only to the federal AKS; thus, organizations should be wary of state-based AKS laws (some of which do not have safe harbors), to which the federal AKS safe harbors do not apply.
3. IRS FS 2011-11, October 20, 2011, Clarification of Notice 2011-20 Q18

SECTION 2

CHAPTER 5

Implementation of Stage II Alignment Models

We have provided you with a comprehensive overview of all the considerations that should go into deciding whether to pursue a CIN and, moreover, what strategy to take once you determine that a Clinically Integrated Network (CIN) is the organization's next step. We will now consider a few ways to implement these strategies.

It is important to understand that many of the functions that are necessary to establish a CIN (i.e., the formation of clinical processes and guidelines, the establishment of quality metrics, etc.) should be reviewed continuously and revised as applicable. These ever-changing foundations should be the ongoing motivation and basis of the CIN. Again, we will focus on the formation of a CIN in this chapter as it is one of the more common (and straightforward) Stage II models, but these same concepts can be applied to all clinically integrated organizations, regardless of the model pursued.

Once the core tenets of the CIN are considered (IT infrastructure, cost accounting, and legal compliance), the organization should seek to establish these components in the most efficient manner possible so the organization can continue to grow and mature. Therefore, the CIN should pursue a care process design system (CPDS) and population health management (PHM) strategy first. Then, the organization should consider all of the payer contracts needed to perform their work and begin renegotiating all of the contracts.

CARE PROCESS DESIGN SYSTEM

The CPDS is essentially the process of retooling the care delivery system via key frontline individuals. The CPDS goes beyond the preliminary, foundation-setting stages of clinical integration and describes a *system* for the transformation stage of clinical integration where value production begins.

CPDS Overview

As Figure 2.5.1 illustrates, the CPDS has four main components. While the subsequent sections explain each component in greater detail, it is important to note that these four parts signify interdependent pieces of the puzzle that, when executed effectively and applied consistently, create a system that allows for care delivery transformation and align with the goals and expected outcomes of a CIN. The primary intent of the CPDS is to develop a model that is both responsive to the existent and upcoming changes in healthcare and beneficial for the organization in multiple ways; therefore, it is a system that can be utilized as the vehicle for implementing the foundations needed to form a CIN.

The CPDS has been developed to be a system, as opposed to a temporary project or initiative; thus, the CPDS represents a critical mental

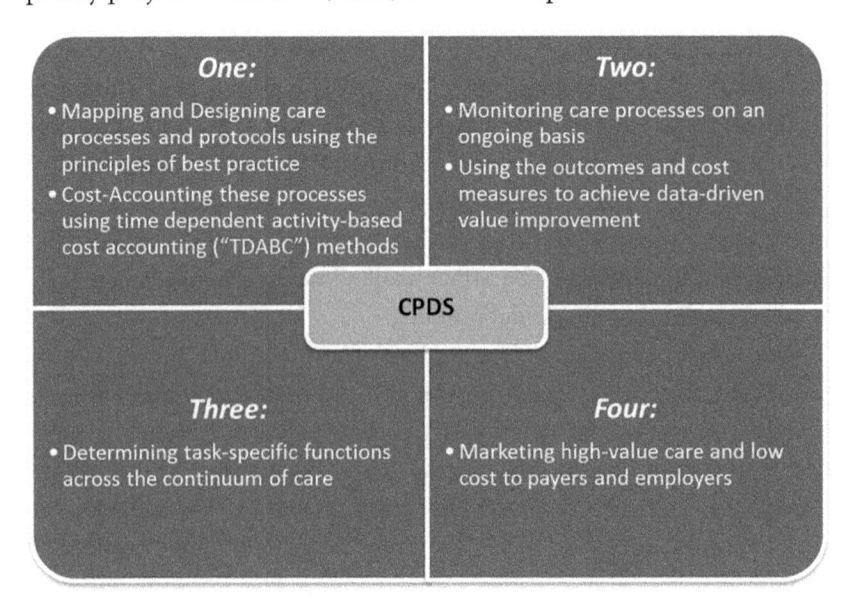

One:
- Mapping and Designing care processes and protocols using the principles of best practice
- Cost-Accounting these processes using time dependent activity-based cost accounting ("TDABC") methods

Two:
- Monitoring care processes on an ongoing basis
- Using the outcomes and cost measures to achieve data-driven value improvement

CPDS

Three:
- Determining task-specific functions across the continuum of care

Four:
- Marketing high-value care and low cost to payers and employers

FIGURE 2.5.1 Basic Components of the CPDS

and cultural shift from the "standard" care delivery process to one that is anchored by the principles of clinical integration. Moreover, the CPDS model requires that the organization already has established a strong provider base that is tied to the organization and one another via the same values, goals, and objectives, with the patient the foundation of a CIN or other clinically integrated organization. The primary reason for this prerequisite is that, once in place, the CPDS will be a permanent part of the organization and vehicle for change. In other words, the CPDS will be the basis for the future of the organization's care delivery process and will serve as the backbone for the organization's brand and market recognition.

By its very nature, the CPDS model is designed to advance the value proposition systematically. As the market and industry continue to sharpen the spotlight on value, the outcomes of the CPDS will allow the CIN to differentiate itself in the marketplace as a high-value producer of healthcare services.

The CPDS model will not be unique to how one service or the other is delivered. Rather, once implemented, it will be the system by which the organization *designs, monitors, and improves* the value of all its services.

The CPDS is adaptable to multiple types of organizations (i.e., hospitals, specific service lines, physician practices, ancillary service providers, post-acute providers, etc.) and is especially useful in implementing the necessary foundations of a CIN. Again, while it applies to both a fee-for-volume and a fee-for-value based reimbursement model, it is particularly useful in organizations such as a CIN, where there is a need for a systematic design of care processes that produce reliably desirable outcomes for quality and cost. Moreover, it is arguably the optimal system for organizations in a combination reimbursement market (i.e., both FFS and FFV), which is likely to be the dominant payment arrangement for most parts of the country over the next three to five years. As we discuss later in this chapter, the CPDS factors in the importance of production and, thus, operates in a manner that derives volume through value through such matters as the creation of more cost-effective care process units.

The CPDS Design Teams

The CPDS system will develop through multidisciplinary design teams comprising physician leaders, clinical and nonclinical experts, financial experts (trained in time-dependent, activity-based cost accounting), process and performance improvement experts (instructed in Lean process care mapping techniques), and patients who have previously undergone the process or procedure under design.

Each CPDS design team will be tasked with mapping and embedding best-practice guidelines into the CIN, relating their experience with the process to the cost accounting experts. The result of this collaborative effort will be a compilation of care maps and associated performance measures and metrics that are representative of the most commonly utilized care processes of the organization.

Physician Leaders

The physician's roles and responsibilities[1] on the design team will include:

- **Leading the team.** In the sense of ensuring the team stays focused on the big picture of moving toward value production (i.e., quality/cost), if the team's physician leader does not endorse this concept, it is highly unlikely that the other members of the team will follow and fully engage in the activities.
- **Lending expertise.** The physician will need to strike a balance between contributing his or her knowledge and experience with the process under consideration and ensuring that others have the opportunity to contribute their thoughts and ideas to the design phase of the team's work. The *integrated* delivery system and the CPDS, particularly in the early development stages, require a collaborative approach to be wholly functional and sustainable.
- **Practicing data-driven value improvement.** Possibly the most important role for the physician will be to monitor the outcomes of the process over time and adjust processes on a continuous basis to ensure that value (quality per unit of cost) remains high.

Process Mapping

While many hospitals and other healthcare organizations are now hiring experts trained in Lean process engineering, the CPDS design teams will only require someone capable of mapping out the key steps in the process using a modified Lean process mapping technique. This technique can be taught to most clinical, and even nonclinical, healthcare workers in a short period and should not be a major obstacle in implementing this system.

Time Dependent, Activity-Based Cost Accounting

Unlike the process mapping, the time-dependent, activity-based cost accounting (TDABC) methodology requires some familiarity with activity-based cost accounting, and most business analysts and others in healthcare financial departments can perform this work. It also does not require purchasing expensive cost accounting software systems. Large hospital systems have done this manually using Microsoft® Excel® spreadsheets.

The main idea here is to apply a methodology that factors in the true costs of care, as opposed to using more nebulous and, thus, less beneficial forms of cost accounting, such as ratios of costs to charges or labor RVUs.[2]

Patients

Lastly, it cannot be emphasized enough how essential it is for the patients to be a part of the CPDS design teams. True patient-centered care cannot be developed without the input of those who recently have experienced care from this perspective. The CPDS team should make every effort to seek out and involve patients in the design process on an ongoing basis.

Best Practice/Evidence-Based Design

It is a common misunderstanding that healthcare delivery includes only practices that are supported by the scientific literature. The truth is that the driver of a vast majority of clinical care is provider preference, habit, or simply "that's the way we've always done it" and not by rigid scientific study.[3] Further, many of the practices in question will never undergo a randomized clinical trial.

Accordingly, the quality and cost outcomes data measurements obtained through the CPDS will provide a way to study the process designs. Further, using objective information to determine what works and what doesn't as an ongoing iterative process continues under the direction of each physician leader.

The Role Of The Healthcare Information Technology

By the time the organization begins to consider the CPDS model, the assumption is that its clinical integration infrastructure has been established or is well underway. The CPDS will rely heavily on a robust information technology (IT) platform, which is a requisite for all CINs. As such, the CIN's IT infrastructure will allow the organization to have the following six capabilities that will lend to its ability to carry out PHM functions:

1. Continuous assessment and monitoring of patient populations;
2. Application of clinical filters to enable risk stratification based on assessments;
3. Use of clinical workflows (best practices) to implement interventions based on risk level and evidence-based medicine;
4. Generation of data based on configured metrics (outcomes and costs);
5. Reporting and sharing of data among all providers and care practitioners involved; and
6. Improvement of the care delivery system and/or intervention based on analysis of data.

As illustrated in Figure 2.5.2, and previously noted, organizations undertaking CPDS development will strive to become true "learning" organizations. Here, the information flow of quality and cost measures

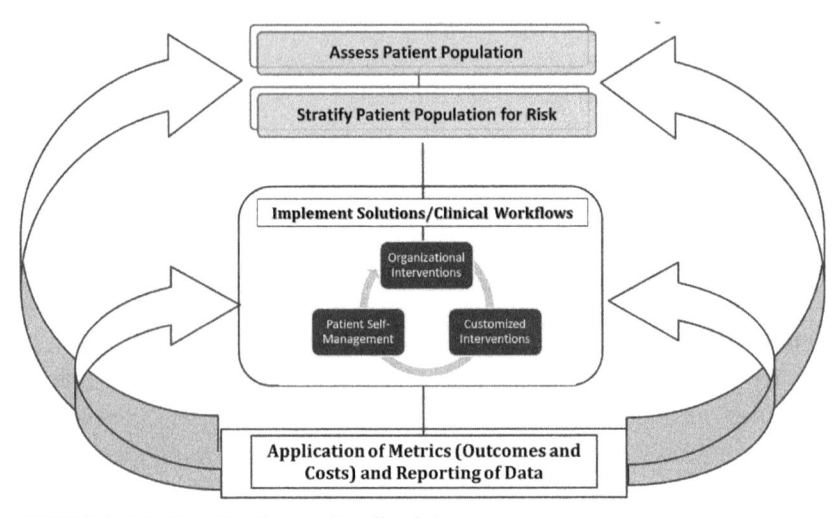

FIGURE 2.5.2 Care Continuum Feedback Loop

within the clinical delivery system is fed back to providers via continuous feedback loops and used to drive ongoing performance improvement and enhanced delivery of value to the healthcare consumer. Then, the knowledge gained from this system will be used to expand the "evidence base" of medical science.

For an organization to be considered a truly clinically integrated, value-based organization, it must have in place a system that can provide its consumers with high-quality and low-cost care. It must demonstrate its ability to generate value, hold its providers accountable for their performance, and gather and apply information in a manner that promotes population health management, as well as process/outcomes improvement. The CPDS offers all of these capabilities and more, making it just the system a progressive organization needs to develop a sustainable, affordable, and valuable care delivery model that can ultimately facilitate its long-term success. In the next section, we will focus more on the population health aspect of this system.

POPULATION HEALTH MANAGEMENT

PHM is a general concept that refers to "health outcomes and their distribution in a population. Here, outcomes are achieved by patterns of health determinants (such as medical care, public health, sociological status, physical environment, individual behavior, and genetics) over the life course" of the population.[4] Essentially, it is the commitment to managing health across the continuum of care for the betterment of a subset of the population. This improvement is a key targeted outcome of value-based reimbursement models as payers seek to incentivize value over volume. Ultimately, PHM will become the primary function for CINs.

The main elements for deriving a successful PHM strategy are to develop information-powered clinical decision making, establish a primary care-led clinical workforce, and induce patient engagement and community integration. To accomplish these goals, organizations should consider the "4M" approach in concert with the CPDS, or as an alternative to that system. The 4M approach is a comprehensive, replicable, and scalable way of retooling the clinical enterprise. While it is similar in many aspects to the CPDS, it is slightly less encompassing and may be more manageable for organizations beginning to experiment with these types of care transformations. It consists of four components: method, measures, mechanisms, and means, and it seeks to help CINs move from volume to value while rewarding providers for their successful transition and transformation into affordable care.

Method

The method is to use a systematic approach to revamping the care delivery toward PHM using multidisciplinary teams comprising frontline clinical and nonclinical caregivers. First, organizations should complete a comprehensive assessment of risks for individuals within the population. Next, PHM resources (i.e., care managers, care providers, integrated care models, etc.) are allocated to the population on an as-needed basis. Specifically, the allocation of the most resources is to the highest risk patients. At that point, the care teams are developed to include an expanded primary care platform that can focus on prevention and wellness of a vast population. This platform is critical as primary care physicians provide the ability to coordinate care across the entire continuum (i.e., health risk assessment, primary prevention, chronic disease management, acute ambulatory care, acute inpatient care, post-acute care, and hospice care).

The teams use an array of techniques to accomplish their care process design activities, including a form of modified Lean care process mapping. Best-practice care guidelines are established for each step in the process, informed by the evidence base and the caregiver's knowledge, experience, and innovative ideas. Also, these best practices should be selectively allocated to the areas of greatest need and over time resources should be reallocated to respond appropriately to those portions of the population who demonstrate the highest need for improvement.

Organizations should seek to establish vigorous measurements of quality and cost outcomes. Specifically, the CIN should measure true outcomes and costs to the organization rather than the payers. This measurement should encompass continuous learning with feedback of outcome data to providers resulting in ongoing data-driven process improvements. Moreover, the CIN should attempt to develop clinical predictive modeling through the application of techniques for sound PHM.

Measures

As noted, it is crucial for organizations to establish clear methods for determining quality, patient satisfaction, and cost efficiency outcomes. Doing so enables an organization to rank providers according to their outcomes measurements, quality, and cost efficiency. High performers receive preferential referrals, and their clinical process and procedures are used to guide best-practice care design. Low performers are motivated to adopt best practices to gain more referrals and improve their ranking.

Further, the CIN should seek to measure the total impact of their PHM initiative. Again, these data will include cost and quality measures such as unnecessary ER visits or readmissions for the entirety of the managed population. Other more population-based metrics should be considered, such as management of chronic conditions (e.g., diabetic adults) and screening protocols (e.g., colorectal and breast cancer). CINs should transform their capabilities and conquer longitudinal metrics, such as per-member-per-month costs. Finally, these measures should seek to determine the population-wide impact on quality of life and functional assessments/effectiveness measures.

Mechanisms

The primary mechanism for implementing a PHM strategy is the inclusion of a robust clinical IT system. This system should include applications to support the care process design system through process mapping and time-driven, activity-based cost accounting (TDABC). Additionally, applications should be established to support the full range of PHM elements and patient outreach and engagement. These patient communications should include, but not be limited to, health risk assessments, patient risk stratification, patient education and awareness, chronic disease management, patient self-care and group learning through social networking, and patient surveys and self-reported outcome measurements. Moreover, patient interaction will continue to evolve to manage patients where they live, both physically and virtually, leading to the use of telemedicine at a level that is even hard to imagine at this stage.

Finally, these applications also should be designed to support care delivery through provider-facing apps. These provider-focused applications should include decision support, information sharing, care guidelines, cost transparency, quality outcomes, education and training, and patient communication.

Means

The final component of the 4M structure is the means by which the CIN can manage risks and maximize the return-on-investment of these changes. Organizations should consider reinsuring the risk through provider-owned insurance captives or development of high-value, narrow networks. Additionally, and as will be discussed more in the next section, CINs should begin participating in value-based risk contracting for these PHM services. The TDABC will be critical for successful pricing and negotiating value-based reimbursements, specifically for models such as shared savings, bundled payments, partial and global capitation with knowledge of true costs, and maintenance of margins.

Once the CIN decides the means of establishing these cost benefits, it must determine how best to predict these financial incentives to budget appropriately and determine where it can realize savings. Moreover, these shared savings will have to be distributed to the various parties appropriately, including the participating providers.

RENEGOTIATION OF PAYER CONTRACTS

The end goal of the CIN is to be able to renegotiate contracts for all participating entities under the integrated model via collective bargaining. Depending on the organization and how fully integrated it becomes, this renegotiation can transpire via a single legal entity or the CIN can be the messenger for all integrated practices. Either way, CINs should be the primary point of contact for all payer contracts, as the Stage II model will allow the consumers to capture higher value. Again, it is critical that organizations broach this once all other portions of the CIN have been formed and matured to ensure that the CIN not only can participate legally in this manner, but also can take advantage of value-based reimbursement models.

Should the CIN be wary of participating in risk-based contracts, the structure still offers a significant advantage for organizations. As discussed multiple times, the CIN (if structured appropriately to meet the legal requirements) will be able to contract on behalf of all the practices and likely will be able to negotiate better contracts as a result. At a minimum, the CIN can reduce some overhead expenses related to negotiating contracts with each practice individually, although this is not the primary nor the targeted result. Additionally, the CIN can provide a vehicle for the organizations to participate in contracts that offer incentives for actions like preventative care, delivery of high-value care, and delivery of cost-efficient care, that have not been incentivized by most payers until now (i.e., value-based contracts).

Organizations should take their time in pursuing fee-for-value contracts, as the complete shift will take some time, and fee-for-service contracts will persist indefinitely. In fact, some fee-for-service contracts likely will remain in perpetuity. As such, there is time for the payers and their participating organizations to determine what needs to be tweaked to create a "win-win-win" scenario between the healthcare organization, the payers, and the patients. CINs will be structured to begin testing these scenarios, but organizations should consider what other players in their market are doing.

Once the CIN has determined the benefit of actively engaging in a value-based reimbursement model, various opportunities become available. Some key examples are shared savings agreements, bundled payments, and even capitation, as we outlined in Chapter 3 of this section. Although this is not necessarily a requirement for the organization, as the industry moves more aggressively toward these models, the Stage II models inherently will be best equipped to participate and reap the benefits. Moreover, these shared savings and incentive payments can then be distributed to the physicians as part of the overall compensation structure, further tying the goals of the organization with the individual motivation of the physicians.

CONCLUSION

The implementation tactics addressed in this chapter vary across the different Stage II alignment models and differing organizations, geographic locations, and sizes. Nevertheless, the basic tenets of each tactic should be considered for all. As the clinically integrated organization is established, the question becomes how best to ensure realized clinical change as opposed to just the legal changes. The options for implementing change successfully are vast and could be combined or built upon, but we tend to recommend the use of the CPDS and the 4M systems as a general structure. Once the implementation is complete, organizations should consider how best to capitalize on these structures via the renegotiation of payer contracts.

These techniques will determine the actual success of the organization, from both a clinical and financial perspective, and they inherently tie together. It is important to understand that just because a Stage II model meets the legal requirements laid out, it may not necessarily demonstrate a clinical impact on the population it serves, which in turn results in minimal positive financial results. Thus, it is imperative that the organization seeks to implement and continuously improve on the clinical changes desired for the organization (i.e., improved quality and patient access, reduction of costs, and the establishment of a continuum of care).

If all of these matters are achieved successfully, there are clear return-on-investment opportunities. First and foremost, the patient satisfaction should increase as the organization responds to their needs and desires while maintaining a high quality of care. Also, organizations can expect to realize a preservation of their margin or enhanced margins via the processes related to cost controls. Moreover, the CIN will be able to capitalize on economies of scale, which will result in a decrease in costs or an overall lower per-member-per-month cost.

As the practices work together, the referral patterns will strengthen, which will increase revenues for the CIN. These referral patterns and the collaboration also will lead to continued overall growth of the CIN's population, resulting in a greater market share for the CIN and potential market dominance. Finally, the Stage II model will see benefits from participating in value-based reimbursement contracts through incentives and shared savings.

A CIN or Stage II alignment model is not the only answer to responding to the changes in the industry that have resulted from the Accountable Care Era, nor is it one we would recommend that every organization pursue. However, if the organization has considered the alternatives carefully and is knowledgeable of the costs and commitment required to participate successfully in such an arrangement, a Stage II alignment model can offer a comprehensive strategy for preparing to engage in a value-based healthcare environment.

REFERENCES

1. Lee TH. Turning doctors into leaders. *Harvard Business Review*. 2010 (April):50-59.; https://hbr.org/2010/04/turning-doctors-into-leaders. Accessed November 9, 2016.
2. Young DW. The folly of using RCCs and RVUs for intermediate product costing. *Health Finance Manage*. 2007;61(4):100-106, 108.; http://www.davidyoung.org/resources/docs/rvu.pdf. Accessed November 9, 2016.
3. Charles C, Gafni A, Freeman E. The evidence-based medicine model of clinical practice: scientific teaching or belief-based preaching? *J Eval Clin Pract*. 2011;17(4):597-605.
4. Kindig D. Understanding population health terminology. *The Milbank Quarterly*. 2007. https://www.ncbi.nlm.nih.gov/pmc/articles/PMC2690307. Accessed November 9, 2016.

SECTION 2

CHAPTER 6

Where Do We Go from Here with Value-Based Structures and Strategies: Will There be a Stage III?

We have outlined in this book how the healthcare industry and more particularly physician practices have utilized different alignment strategies and compensation models to respond to changes in the healthcare marketplace.

RECENT EVOLUTION AND CHANGE

We noted that the historical predominance of volume-based, fee-for-service reimbursements has led to the current situation where most physicians, whether in private practice or as part of an employed network, are compensated for production, as measured by factors like patient visits, hours of work, or work relative value units (wRVUs).

As the system moves inexorably toward a more value-based, fee-for-value reimbursement environment, we noted that newer alignment vehicles, such as accountable care organizations (ACOs), clinically integrated networks (CINs), and patient-centered medical homes (PCHMs) are beginning to take shape. Also, more and more physician compensation models now include at least partial incentives for performance, as measured by such matters as specialty-specific quality metrics, cost efficiency metrics, meaningful use of electronic health records, and other parameters.

The question now becomes, where will the system move from here? Will there be a third generation of physician compensation formulae and alignment vehicles, or will the current second-generation models remain stable for the indefinite future?

To answer this question, we need first to drill down and understand the forces behind seismic shifts in the ways physicians are paid and how they align with other providers to deliver services. None of the major changes that we are now seeing play out in the "reformed" healthcare environment are happening in a vacuum; instead, they represent a definite response to this impetus for change.

The overarching imperative in the healthcare industry today is for the quality of care to improve and for costs of care to decrease, or at least to inflate at a rate more commensurate with the economy as a whole.

The quality of care has been an issue in the U.S. healthcare system since 1999, when the Institute of Medicine (IOM) released its sentinel findings that nearly 100,000 patients die annually as a result of avoidable medical errors in American hospitals. Until that time, most providers, and indeed most patients, were convinced that the quality of care in the U.S. healthcare system was second to none. This, despite the fact that the United States was ranked last for many years before 1999 among economically developed countries on measures of population health quality, such as infant mortality rates, life expectancy, and incidence of chronic disease.

As a result of the IOM report, many initiatives were launched around healthcare quality and patient safety. The Institute for Healthcare Improvement (IHI), in particular, led the charge around attempts to make the hospital environment a safer place. The Centers for Medicare and Medicaid Services (CMS), The Joint Commission (TJC), and others instituted regulatory standards to push hospitals and outpatient facilities toward participation in these programs and compliance with regulatory requirements.

Unfortunately, almost two decades after the IOM report, these efforts have not shown significant results. In fact, a repeat of the IOM study in 2014 revealed that the death toll related to avoidable medical mistakes was up to 400,000 per year and continuing to trend upward.

The cost of healthcare has also become more and more of an issue since the beginning of the 21st century. Particularly in times of economic recession, as experienced in 2008 and 2009, the federal government has demonstrated bipartisan intolerance of the inflationary cost curve related to healthcare spending. This concern played a significant role in the passage of the Affordable Care Act (ACA) in 2010 and subsequent passage of the Medicare Authorization and CHIP Reauthorization Act (MACRA) in 2015. Both of these pieces of legislation included multiple mechanisms by which payment reform was to drive healthcare reform and produce a more value-based care delivery system. While it is too early to tell whether the cost-controlling components of MACRA will work, it is important to note that this law, unlike the ACA, was passed with bipartisan support, and even if the ACA were to be repealed or significantly modified, the overarching goal of controlling costs while maintaining quality will persist.

Therefore, it can be logically predicted that the push for higher value production by the healthcare system will persist over the indefinite future and second generation, value-based organizational structures, and physician compensation models will continue to become more the norm over the indefinite future.

WHERE DO WE GO FROM HERE?

The question of whether this will be the end of the line or whether third generation models will emerge is much harder to predict. However, several forces are now brewing within the industry that will make further evolution into third generation structures and beyond very likely. These dynamics include the following:

1. **The Move toward Population Health Management.** As has been stated many times in this book and elsewhere, achieving the Triple Aim of healthcare delivery (high-quality individual patient care, population health management, and cost control) will be the ultimate goal for providers going forward. The system, however, is not yet ideally structured to deliver true population health management (PHM) services. These services will require additions to the current delivery system, such as the development of a comprehensive IT infrastructure that allows for the virtual provision of health risk assessments and remote delivery of care management, and even acute medical services. In addition, the best reimbursement and provider compensation models will need to be determined for PHM

services. Capitated reimbursements are likely to play a prominent role in this regard; however, it has yet to be determined if other reimbursement models, such as bundled payments for chronic disease management over periods of time, might also be utilized. The organizational structures that will house PHM are also yet to be determined and may include traditional models of care delivery. Examples include closed staff clinic models or extremely novel organizations, such as online, virtual care networks that span local, regional, or even national geographies.
2. **Virtual Care Delivery.** As described above regarding PHM, healthcare delivery is likely to be rendered virtually in the future via the Internet and all manner of mobile technologies. It is likely that these innovative care channels also will involve unique and novel reimbursement mechanisms. Clayton Christenson, one of the foremost thought leaders in healthcare innovation, has described the use of social networks in the management of chronic diseases, suggesting subscriptions to such networks, where both healthcare professionals and patients can communicate with each other and help or advise those afflicted with similar chronic illnesses to better manage their conditions.
3. **The Persistence of Fee-for-Service Medicine.** While much of the conversation around first- or second-generation care delivery or reimbursement models emphasize the move from volume to value, most seasoned observers of the healthcare economy believe that fee-for-service payments will never disappear from the marketplace and that some services, such as acute episodic care, likely will always be reimbursed in this fashion. Likewise, hospitals probably will continue to be the preferred venue for treating acutely ill patients. Further, while it is expected that going forward more and more care will be delivered in the ambulatory care arena, those with critical illnesses are apt always to require the kind of care that can only be rendered in an inpatient facility.
4. **Reorganization of Primary and Specialty Care Providers.** Expectations are that third generation models for organizing and compensating providers of healthcare services will differ between primary care and specialty care practitioners. Prospectively, primary care increasingly will assume PHM responsibilities and be paid in a capitated fashion for maintaining the health of large populations

of patients. Specialty care providers, on the other hand, are apt to be paid via a bundled or fee-for-service payment mechanism for rendering care to individual patients who suffer from acute episodic illnesses or need acute procedural interventions.

5. **Consolidation of Providers and Payers.** We already see a rash of mergers and acquisitions within the healthcare industry. Hospitals and healthcare systems continue to acquire scores of physician practices and organize them into integrated delivery networks (IDNs). Many hospitals and healthcare systems also are merging or being acquired by larger systems. A similar process is ongoing in the payer realm where many commercial insurers are consolidating into larger regional or national companies. Finally, government payers are playing a greater role in healthcare reimbursement systems. Some believe that this will ultimately result in a single-payer or universal health system run by the government and similar to what we see in many other economically developed countries. Obviously, consolidating payers and providers in this way would result in organizational and economic structures yet unseen in the American healthcare system. One need only look to the national health services in countries like Great Britain and Canada to get an idea of how radically such a move would change the landscape of the U.S. healthcare system.

6. **Regulatory Reforms.** It is hard to overstate the degree to which legal regulations mandate the way in which providers deliver healthcare in the United States. Currently hospitals and healthcare systems must ascribe to a number of arcane rules regarding the self-referral of patients or the kick-back of fees when designing provider compensation models. Newer, government-sponsored, provider organizations, such as Medicare ACOs, include waivers that exempt eligible providers from having to comply with these regulations. It will be interesting to see if other novel provider organizations, such as commercial CINs, primary or specialty care medical homes, or all-payer population health models, such as the Comprehensive Primary Care Plus (CPC +) program, will also include these waivers and slowly decrease the regulatory burden under which providers in the healthcare industry now have to operate. It does not take much imagination to envision how the lifting of some of these regulations could dramatically change the way providers are organized or compensated in the future.

7. **The Elimination of Third-Party Payers.** As we've seen, third-party payers determine many of the rules and regulations regarding healthcare reimbursements. In fact, many believe that eliminating this element of the healthcare marketplace, by having providers directly contract with employers or individuals, would benefit the system by eliminating non-value-added administrative costs and unleashing provider-based innovations. The move toward direct to employer or individual contracting may be accelerated by a growing sense of consumerism now present in the healthcare system, wherein high-deductible or so-called self-directed healthcare plans are becoming more and more prevalent. How far this type of reimbursement will go and how many providers or consumers will choose to forgo the use of third-party intermediaries is yet to be seen; however, this possibility must be considered as we attempt to forecast the course of future change in the system.

CONCLUSION

In summary, the significant changes we have seen and are currently witnessing within the healthcare system are primarily driven by the overarching goals of the system to improve quality of care and lower costs.

As the system evolves into organizational and compensation structures that are designed to improve value (quality/cost), it is interesting to contemplate where we go from here and whether third generation and beyond models are on the horizon and if we can anticipate even more change in the way doctors are organized and paid within the system.

Several factors may bring about future changes in the system. One is the commitment by many in the system to achieve the so-called Triple Aim of healthcare delivery, especially to improve the health of populations cared for by a system that may be more consolidated, less regulated, and more innovative and responsive to the demands of those it is intended to serve.